THERE'S **NO** manual

THERE'S NO MANUAL

Honest + Gory Wisdom

ABOUT HAVING A BABY

BETH NEWELL AND JACKIE ANN RUIZ

ILLUSTRATIONS BY JACKIE ANN RUIZ

AVERY | AN IMPRINT OF PENGUIN RANDOM HOUSE | NEW YORK

AVERY

an imprint of Penguin Random House LLC

penguinrandomhouse.com

Most Avery books are available at special quantity discounts for bulk purchase for sales promotions, premiums, fund-raising, and educational needs. Special books or book excerpts also can be created to fit specific needs. For details, write SpecialMarkets@penguinrandomhouse.com.

Library of Congress Cataloging-in-Publication Data

Names: Newell, Beth, author. | Ruiz, Jackie Ann, author.
Title: There's no manual : honest and gory wisdom about having a baby /
Beth Newell and Jackie Ann Ruiz ; illustrations by Jackie Ann Ruiz.
Description: New York : Avery, an imprint of Penguin Random House, [2020] |
Includes bibliographical references and index. |
Identifiers: LCCN 2019038403 (print) | LCCN 2019038404 (ebook) |
ISBN 9780525534358 (trade paperback) | ISBN 9780525534365 (epub)
Subjects: LCSH: Pregnancy—Popular works. | Childbirth—Popular works.
Classification: LCC RG525 .N42 2020 (print) | LCC RG525 (ebook) | DDC 618.2—dc23
LC record available at https://lccn.loc.gov/2019038403
LC ebook record available at https://lccn.loc.gov/2019038404

p.   cm.

Printed in the United States of America

1 3 5 7 9 10 8 6 4 2

Book design by Lorie Pagnozzi

Neither the publisher nor the authors are engaged in rendering professional advice or services to the individual reader. The ideas, procedures, and suggestions contained in this book are not intended as a substitute for consulting with your physician. All matters regarding your health require medical supervision. Neither the authors nor the publisher shall be liable or responsible for any loss or damage allegedly arising from any information or suggestion in this book.

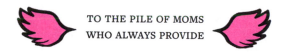 TO THE PILE OF MOMS
WHO ALWAYS PROVIDE

CONTENTS

THERE'S **NO** manual

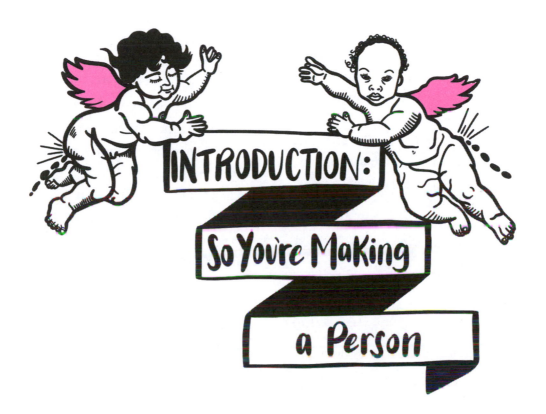

INTRODUCTION:
So You're Making
a Person

INTRODUCTION

> New moms and pregnant women are
> bombarded with unsolicited advice
> from every direction. We hear it from
> our family, friends, coworkers, the
> internet, and that unhappy-looking
> woman in our apartment building
> who keeps telling us to put a hat on
> the baby before he catches a cold.
> In August. With so much conflicting
> advice, it's hard to know who to
> listen to. Here's our advice: fuck
> advice.

There's no real manual for motherhood—except this one.

Other books will tell you how to make your ascent into motherhood a streamlined, predictable process, of nap "time," sleep "training," and feeding "schedules." Not only is it impossible to live up to all that advice, but surrounding ourselves with a series of boxes to check gives women an entirely misleading idea of what's in store for them. The reality of bringing life into the world involves exhaustion, pain, tears, and so much milk, spilled, splattered, and spewed all over everything you own. And there are moments when you're awake in the middle of the night—tiredly nursing your baby while you google photos of newborn rash—that you feel totally helpless and alone, in spite of all your preparation and research.

But you also get to be a literal goddess, capable of creating human life, which is pretty cool. No one talks much about that part either.

This having-a-baby thing is hard. And not in the "ha ha, diapers are really stinky, oh boy, I am not ready to be a father" way you've seen portrayed in the movies. Like really hard, in a gut-twisting, bone-shifting, perineal-tearing way that is impossible to fully convey to anyone who hasn't crawled through the baby trenches. It's hard enough as it is down here "in the shit." Don't add to that stress by trying to perform motherhood to other people's standards and regimens. Instead, focus on survival. And laughter. That's what we're aiming to help you with in this book. Don't get us wrong—many of those other parenting books are filled with gems of wisdom—but we want to cut the BS and give it to you straight—the way your best friend would. We're here to tell you that those early days of parenting might include as much sobbing into a pillow about your boobs and the fact that your husband doesn't have any as it does staring lovingly at your newborn. That's normal.

And it's normal to have pregnancy and baby problems that bear no resemblance to your friend's pregnancy and baby problems.

It's also normal to confuse your baby's first fetal movements with fart bubbles. And it's normal to confuse your early contractions with bad gas. A lot of this mom stuff is confusing and farty, but don't worry—you'll get through this. We wrote this book while our babies were letting out some pretty distracting ass burps (please forgive the tupos). We can do anything. Women are fucking magic.

APOLOGIES IN ADVANCE

This book is meant to help you get through all the difficulties of having a baby. But it will not do justice to what some go through. That group includes, but is not limited to: single mothers, mothers of color, women undergoing in vitro fertilization, adoptive parents, surrogates, trans men carrying babies, mothers carrying multiples, and mothers suffering miscarriages or other health issues. We wanted to speak to the common burdens of pregnancy and childbirth, which we felt were not being fully represented in popular literature. We hope you get something out of this, and that somewhere a tired mom is finding a way to speak to the issues we were unable to cover. We see you, and we support you.

ONE MORE NOTE
BEFORE WE BEGIN

This book is divided up into sections, but we recommend reading it all at once. You may think now, "I'll read that part once the baby arrives," but trust us, you won't. You'll be too tired. There's lots of stuff that'll be easier to emotionally and physically prepare for in advance rather than in the moment. You won't need all of this info, but we want you to make the most of what's helpful. You can always skim now and refer back later. You got this!

A BRIEF HISTORY OF BIRTH UNTIL NOW

On our journey to try to tell you everything that everyone forgot to tell you about having a kid, we may as well start at the beginning of human procreation, with a brief history of how women have been making life with their bodies.

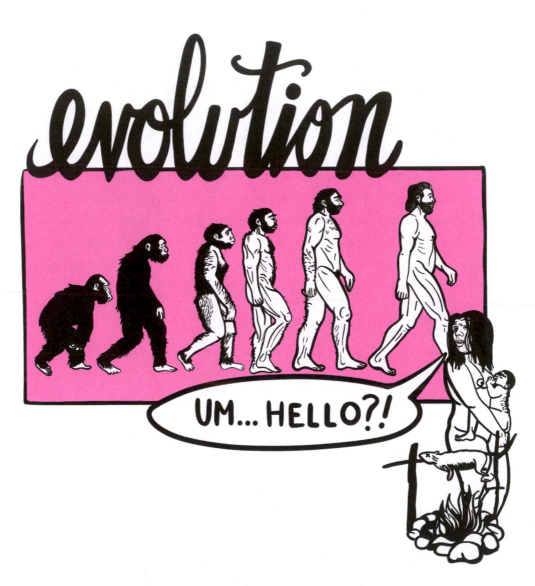

160,000 BC — A *Homo erectus* woman births the first *Homo sapiens* baby. While she doesn't have the language or ability to recognize his larger brain, she does note to herself that "Fuck, this head is huge," and "This one seems needy." Evolution charts will later write women out of the story of evolution, depicting man's emergence as a feat unto himself, with hairy apes and men striding confidently across time into existence, their tired cave wives forgotten.

160,000 BC to 320 BC — Women continue to make humanity happen, largely unnoticed, while men make large sculptures of their dicks and other dicklike objects.

320 BC — The first known cesarean section is performed in the birth of Indian emperor Bindusara. Concerned parties immediately question whether the baby's survival was "natural" enough.

Zeroish — Mary wants to have a home birth but is thwarted by societal pressures.

1500s to 1800s — Men start to enter the field of midwifery in order to show women how they've been doing it wrong. They begin "helping" with painful medical advances, including episiotomies and forceps.

1865 — Lifesaving baby formula is invented by a German dude. Women are immediately shamed for using it.

1881 — Nitrous oxide, or laughing gas, is used for the first time to treat labor pain. The United States quickly disregards this effective, controllable, and noninvasive treatment, deciding that it is better suited to countries where women's health and well-being are a higher priority.

1900s — Medical schools change the name of midwifery to obstetrics, because it sounds "smarter" and "less girly."

1909 — Epidurals are introduced as a pain-relief option during labor, with women immediately questioning whether they deserve them.

1914 — Doctors introduce medicated "twilight sleep" to give mothers the gift of having no memory of meeting their babies.

1950s — With the rising quality of life, more and more women gain the "freedom" to focus on being moms 24-7.

1970s — Ina May Gaskin begins a new "natural birth" movement, which quickly turns into a way for women to judge one another while we navigate the mess men have made.

1996 to 2010 — C-section rates rise dramatically because OBs want to get home and watch *The Sopranos.*

2020 — This book is published. Everything is fixed. Women will never judge one another for making decisions based off their own individual circumstances again.

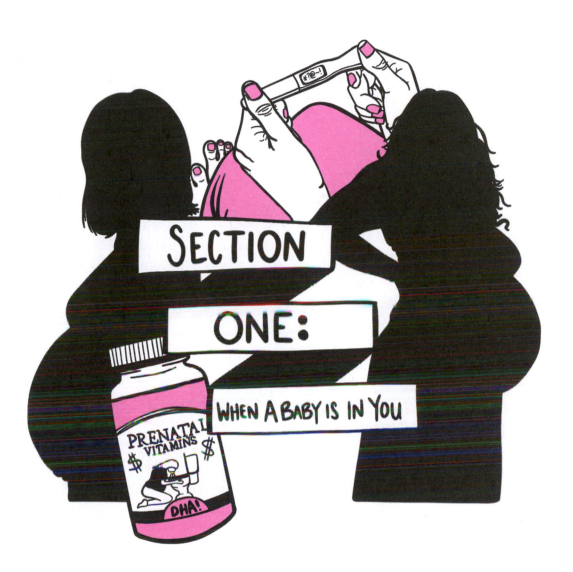

WEIRD SYMPTOMS THAT MIGHT MEAN YOU'RE PREGNANT

So, to start off, congrats! You're pregnant! Or are you? Because pregnancy is like nothing else your body has done, all the symptoms are very weird and vague! Here's what the early stage might feel like.

YOU'VE BEEN BARFING A BIT, OR MORE THAN A BIT

Some women don't barf, and some women do it all day every day. But any amount of regular vomming is terrible, so if it's happening to you, we're here to say "Fuuuck that!" in your honor and also "Congrats on being pregnant!" Talk to your health-care provider if nausea is severe.

YOU'RE HUNGRY *AND* WANT TO BARF

Do you feel nauseous? Or hungry? Or a strange combination of both? Are you violently craving a hamburger just minutes after retching over the toilet? Is there a vague feeling of badness that haunts your digestive system? Anything weird regarding your appetite is a possible symptom of pregnancy.

EVERYTHING SMELLS AND TASTES VERY, VERY BAD

The smell and taste of certain things may make you want to crawl out of your own skin. This heightened sensitivity of your body's lizard brain is trying to save you from eating poison-y stuff. Things you've always found gross, like your partner's morning breath, might make you gag. And formerly innocuous favorites, like seafood or Cheetos, will suddenly seem rancid. You may also find yourself asking "Is something burning?" when someone lights a match two blocks away. Avoid what you can and try to appreciate your superhuman abilities despite picking up the distinct floral bouquet of every stranger's BO.

YOU HAVE CRAMPS BUT NOT PERIOD CRAMPS

Experiencing some intense cramping at the wrong time of the month? These wake-you-up-in-the-night pains could be the first signs of an embryo burrowing into your uterine lining. Yep, it's weird, and you're feeling it!

YOU'RE SPOTTING SPOTTING

I spy with my little eye something that is light bleeding that ranges from pink to red to brown! Is a mystery unfolding in your undies? This is just your first taste of the coming grossness of pregnancy!

YOU'RE DROOLING?

Are you walking around like an excited dog on a hot day? Slurring like a college student on her birthday? That's the old mom-to-be drool mouth! Just another totally natural and beautiful part of pregnancy gifted by the goddess as you re-up on the cycle of life.

YOU'RE THIRSTIER THAN A CAMEL AT ITS EX'S WEDDING

You'll need to drink a lot of water to sustain the new increased blood volume in your body and, eventually, the amniotic fluid. Have at it. And if water bores you, try decaf teas. Just be sure to look up possible side effects of any herbal ingredients. For example, licorice root, in certain quantities, can induce premature labor.

YOU'RE A LITTLE . . . BACKED UP

Can't remember the last time you pooped? Progesterone increases in the first trimester, relaxing smooth muscles to prevent your uterus from contracting prematurely. Unfortunately, your digestive tract is also made up of smooth muscle, and digestion becomes sluggish. Prenatal vitamins with iron can make constipation even worse, so talk to your health-care provider/witch about taking magnesium supplements and try to eat more fiber even though just reading those words makes you want to yak. If you're new to constipation, you'll learn that the stagnation of your body's waste system can also cause headaches, fatigue, and bloating, which adds an extra element of "blah" to your overall "blech" pregnancy feeling. Fun!

YOU'VE RECENTLY FALLEN ASLEEP IN PUBLIC

Tired? Like "can't move" tired? You should be. You're trying to replicate your species. So yeah, if it feels like the weight of the world rests on your uterus, it does. NO PRESSURE.

YOUR TITS ARE ON FIRE

Is your bra no longer enough to contain you? Feeling swollen, sore, or oddly tingly in your boobies? That's Mother Nature tapping your boobs on the shoulder, telling them, "It's your time to shine!"

YOU FEEL FAINT, LIKE A DELICATE LADY

Did you faint like a damsel in distress? Dizzy just from standing? A classic sign of pregnancy is being adorably devoid of oxygen in your brain. Your body is prioritizing blood flow to your babe over blood flow to the rest of you, which is a nice metaphor for your immediate future.

YOUR BRAIN IS A LITTLE BROKEN

If you walk through your week with a vague feeling of "Ummm, what?" it's probably because you have fifteen to forty times the usual amount of progesterone and estrogen sloshing around in your head.

YOU HAVE A PERMANENT HEADACHE

Yep, this too. Sorry.

YOUR STINK HAS CHANGED

Does your armpit smell like someone else's all of a sudden? That's because you're actually two people mixed together now! Congrats.

YOU JUST FEEL EHHHHH . . .

So there's this feeling, probably an extension of morning sickness, where you just feel a wave of badness throughout your body. It's almost metallic or acidic, like you're tasting a battery. It's also kind of like your juice is being sucked from your bones and replaced with shittier juice. If you're pregnant, you might know what the hell we're talking about.

YOU HAVE *ALL* THE FEELINGS

As your hormones quickly ramp up, you may find yourself crying at every commercial, any mention of a commercial, or the memory of a commercial you once saw.* It will seem irrational because it *is* irrational. But also you are entitled to feel this way, so anyone telling you you're being irrational can go to hell. C'mere. We wanna give you a hug. Hug this book. It's gonna be okay.

---

* OMG, remember that T-Mobile commercial at the airport arrivals gate where everyone is singing and hugging? No, *you're* crying!

YOU *LOVE* YOUR PARTNER INTENSELY AND ALSO YOU *HATE* YOUR PARTNER INTENSELY

Normally your PMS week makes you want to claw his eyes out, but suddenly you get all weird and gooey when he walks into a room? You're probably knocked up. If you usually feel pretty good about him but suddenly his every word fills you with Medusa-like rage, you're also probably knocked up. Hormones are responsible for attracting us to a suitable mate, and yours are bonkers now; good luck!

YOUR BASAL BODY TEMPERATURE IS UP

What are you, a little self-monitoring scientist? As if we need to tell you what's going on here, nerd!

YOU JUST *KNOW*

When you know, you know. Do you?

THE PREGNANCY TEST IS POSITIVE!

This is one of the surest signs of pregnancy. If you haven't yet, schedule a visit with your health-care provider.

. . . .

We hope you don't have *all* of these symptoms, but if you do, remember, many of these annoying symptoms are actually a sign that your pregnancy is healthy. You got this!

HOLY SHIT, THIS IS HAPPENING!

Whether your pregnancy is planned or unplanned,* the decision to go forward with having a baby can be described only as a feeling of "Eeeeep!"† You're on a roller coaster you've never ridden, struggling with a complicated safety buckle while the ride has already started moving forward. Here's how to hold it together as you begin the truly wild ride of motherhood.

BREATHE IN SOME FOOD

Take a deep breath and relax. Breathing not your style? Try breathing in a sleeve of cookies or a plate of nachos. Seriously, we're not telling anyone. We're all doing our best, and sometimes our best involves finding comfort in not-so-healthy places. Balance is key, so maybe throw in a banana and some peanut butter to ease your newly discovered mom guilt. As you inhale each cookie, try holding in a crumb-filled breath for a count of one-two-three and slowly release—that's meditating!

REMEMBER: NO ONE KNOWS WHAT THE FUCK THEY'RE DOING

That blissed-out mommy in your prenatal yoga class? She's secretly nervous as fuck. Your friend with multiple kids who somehow seems pretty together? Bedtime makes her want to walk into the sea. The Zen-as-fuck woman teaching your birth class went over her time in therapy last week, after accidentally feeding her nine-month-old honey. No one is 100 percent on top of things and you're certainly not the stupidest person to ever parent, so cut yourself some slack. You're reading this book, so you're already in pretty good shape.

TRY NOT TO IMAGINE EVERY WORST-CASE SCENARIO

It's easy to imagine what could go wrong—in your pregnancy, your birth, your entire child's life. We will all fuck this up a little at some point, and things will still be okay. Sometimes there's nothing we can do but make the best of a bad situation. You're human. You're expected to be human, despite what the parenting literature may imply. Focus on the things you can control. Did we mention breathing in some food?

---

* Yes, we know—"unplanned" sounds a little insulting, as if the majority of pregnancies throughout all of human history were planned! LOLOLOL.

† Also sometimes "OMG," "Ugh," "Wow," or "Oh . . ."

DO FIELD RESEARCH

Pregnancy can turn you into a little anthropologist, observing and interrogating all the other moms. Like a hunter stalking her prey, you'll clock that new mom's every move. Your not-so-secret plan is to hold her down and siphon all of her mom experience directly into your brain. While you're parasiting the knowledge of other moms, try to get a range of opinions. For every woman who vomited every second of her pregnancy, there's a woman who gained eighty pounds. And while neither of those things is medically ideal, they are not always within our control.

REMEMBER THE LIMITS OF ANECDOTAL EVIDENCE

Take everyone's stories with a grain of salt and try not to internalize another woman's negative experience. Also, don't measure yourself too harshly against the healthiest, happiest mom you know. Your experience will be your own, with its own surprises and frustrations, and you'll want to have as positive an attitude as possible. But don't go too far in the opposite direction and tell yourself, "Lisa is crazy. Pregnancy won't be that stressful for *me*." Self-righteousness and overly high expectations will *always* bite you in the ass. This shit is haaaaaaard (we would have added more a's to that word, but we

have a page limit here). It might not be hard for you in the same way it was for Lisa, but it will be hard. Stay positive but be realistic, and bring Lisa an iced coffee next time you see her. Lisa is tired.

IGNORE EVERYONE WHO HAD A BABY MORE THAN A YEAR AGO

People's memories are bad. Don't trust *anyone* who hasn't just been through this. They are looking at this through the nostalgic fog of time. Also they don't want to scare you, so they will openly lie. Trust the woman who just ran through the cross fire. Despite that crazed look in her eyes, *she* remembers. Take her advice. The rest are liars. LIARS!

ACKNOWLEDGE THE PATRIARCHY'S ROLE

Listen. The world will have a lot of opinions about how you should "do" motherhood, and part of your new job is to identify which expectations are put upon you by the patriarchy and which are worth giving a fuck about. If something feels oppressive, trust that. We are in this to build a better world for our tiny babies, and the patriarchy isn't going to fuck itself, after all.

LET YOURSELF GET PSYCHED— YOU GOT THIS!

You're going to have a baby! That's pretty cool. You're going from being a person who, despite a lack of familial obligations, probably ordered delivery four nights this week to a person who is finding the strength to keep a tiny human alive by ordering delivery four nights a week. You're resourceful. You will find new reserves to draw on in order to get this done. And on the other side of all this being there for another person, you will have someone who is there for you, who might also inherit your good cheekbones.

WHEN YOUR LITTLE ONE IS AN OOPSIE

Sometimes, it doesn't matter that you've only had sex once in the past month and you "didn't even orgasm, WTF!" Unplanned pregnancies are *common*. So common, in fact, that the whole world will want to ask you about yours.

"WAS THIS A PLANNED PREGNANCY?"

Until the first time someone asks you this, you'll think, "This cannot be a thing that people think is okay to ask a human woman." Remember, you're pregnant now, and your body is not your own. It legally belongs partly to your growing fetus and apparently to everyone who interacts with you.

Your weapon against most bullshit is always a quick and perfect response, but that rarely happens organically because life is not TV and we can't all be Lorelai Gilmore. In real life, when someone surprises you with a rude question that invades your privacy, it's more likely that you'll think of exactly what to say thirty seconds after the conversation is over. Let's plan ahead. There are many ways to respond to people like this, and we'll list them here, starting with the blunt and ending cordially:

"Are you asking me if my partner deposited his semen inside of me on purpose or by accident?"

Repeating their question back to them is a shortcut to the heart of the matter: *That's none of your fucking business.*

"Was this a planned question, or did you just blurt it out without thinking?"

This is great if you never want to talk to this person again but want them to know that you're smart and witty and they will miss you.

"I'm very happy to be pregnant!"

Raise one eyebrow and kiss their hand; leave immediately. Great for confusing and distracting a person, so you can exit the situation.

"Yeah, the plan is to have a girl, but we'll see; we might change our minds and have a boy!"

Pretending to mishear the question and also pretending not to understand how pregnancy works; the ol' one-two punch. This move will likely produce stunned silence, the perfect time to sashay the fuck away from this annoying person.

"No, it was not a planned pregnancy, but we're very happy to be having a baby."

It takes two people to make a condom break, and women shoulder far too much of the stigma associated with accidental pregnancy. Tell those bitches you got knocked up by accident because you have regular sex with your hot partner and sometimes it's just too hot and the condom breaks. Whoops, your bad for having a great life.

· · · · · · · ·

In some ways, accidental pregnancy really is the perfect segue into parenthood; it's immersion therapy into a new reality where your best-laid plans really don't matter at all. Babies are messy and unpredictable, and they're also full of unexpected joy, just like your new reality. We decided to write this book shortly after both getting accidentally pregnant at the same time, so who knows what doors will open for you because of this careless sexual encounter!

HIDING IT

There are many reasons to keep a pregnancy quiet. Maybe you're trying not to jeopardize a promotion. Maybe you don't want to experience a miscarriage publicly. Or maybe you're just not in the mood for everyone's tales of morning sickness. Whatever the reason, here are some ideas on how to appear not pregnant when you're constantly nauseous and blatantly sober.

TELL PEOPLE YOU'RE SICK

A sick person has every excuse to look nauseous and not drink. It's not contagious anymore, so you came out tonight in order to be interrogated about being visibly miserable!

TELL PEOPLE YOU'RE DOING A DRY JANUARY AND FEBRUARY AND MARCH

Sometimes the only way to convince people you're not pregnant is to act like you actually have a drinking problem.

SAY YOU'RE TRYING A WEIRD NEW DIET

This will explain not only your crankiness but also why you're mostly just eating crackers and vitamins. The latest dieting trend is bread. You heard it on NPR.

TELL EVERYONE YOU'RE SICK *AGAIN*

"You sure have been sick a lot lately," people will say.

"Yes, that's right," you'll say. "It's just one of those summers."

NEVER GO ANYWHERE

Simply avoid bars, restaurants, parties, and basically everywhere your friends are hanging out and having fun. You may feel horribly isolated, but you'll avoid someone asking, "Wait, why aren't you drinking? *Ohmygod,* are you pregnant?!" while you do a terrible job of looking astounded by that question.

ORDER A MOCKTAIL, AND ACT LIKE YOU'RE DRUNK ALREADY

This is apparently what everyone needs from you in order to relax?

· · · · · · · ·

If all else fails, and everyone does start asking, "Wait, are you pregnant?" Tell them, "Yes, but please don't tell anyone! It's still a secret." Everyone in the room will know, but at least Marissa will stop asking you why you won't have "just one glass" of wine.

A "HEALTHY" PREGNANCY

With all its symptoms, the term "healthy pregnancy" sounds like a misnomer. And it's hard to make healthy choices when you have every excuse to chug milkshakes and live on your couch. You're exhausted, you have heartburn, and you're making a goddamn person with your body—so maybe you've earned a third hamburger, *okay?!* Still, you want the person inside of you to get the nutrients they need and exit your body without completely destroying it, so you should probably try to take *some* care of yourself. Here's how to put in the minimal effort.

EAT A PROTEIN AND A VEGETABLE

Despite the traditional wisdom of munching saltines, eating exclusively carbs will actually make your body feel more like crap. Small, frequent protein helps stabilize blood sugar swings, which contribute to nausea. So grab a handful of nuts or a spoonful of nut butter. Leafy greens will help keep your energy up, so sneak them into a smoothie or whatever sort of healthy thing you can stomach. Think of it less as forcing yourself to eat vegetables and more like forcing your child to eat vegetables. And don't worry, we won't make you justify any "bad" decisions. Remember when we said this was about survival?

MOVE A LITTLE

Sure, you *could* continue running[*] during much of pregnancy. But how 'bout just trying to get up off the couch? For every snack you ask your partner to get you, get up and get one yourself. Find the most appealing and easy exercise routine you can, like using the stationary bike on the lowest setting while you rewatch every season of *Drag Race*. Pregnancy's a great time to learn to respect your body's limits. Remember what Mama Ru says: "If you can't love yourself, how in the hell you gonna love somebody else?"

Now is a great time to sign up for a prenatal yoga class, if stretching sounds like it would feel good. These classes are safe for all

---

[*] Depending on your health and previous athletic experience, you may be able to continue running and other activities. But talk to your provider and listen to your body as your pregnancy progresses. And remember to shut up about it around other tired pregnant women.

STRETCHHH!

SAFE + EASY YOGA POSES FOR YOUR CROWDED + ACHING BODY (ALSO GREAT FOR EARLY LABOR!)

On inhale, roll shoulders back, lift chest and head, and let your belly hang. This is **COW POSE**

On exhale, round your spine up toward the ceiling, and drop your head toward your chest. This is **CAT POSE**

CAT/COW

GREAT FOR:
- Low back pain
- "Making room" in your crowded body
- Back labor pain relief

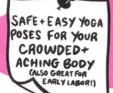

O...

Hands are shoulder-width apart

...MG.

Knees are hip-width apart

BUTTERFLY

GREAT FOR:
- Low back pain
- Tight hip-flexors
- Realizing you need a pedicure

OH HEY, LOOK AT THAT! I DO STILL HAVE TOES!

CHILD'S POSE

GREAT FOR:
- Resting + relieving belly weight for a sec
- Drooling on your mat.

RELAX YR FACE!

Begin by kneeling on a mat or carpet, and sit back to rest your butt on your feet, with knees wide enough to leave space for your belly. Slowly, bring your chest down to the floor, allowing your body to sink between your legs. Extend your arms overhead, resting your forearms, palms, and forehead on the floor. Breathe. Sink. Fart.

Sit up nice + tall, and use your hands to reach behind and pull the flesh of your butt cheeks out of the way, so you're sitting on your sitz bones. Bend your knees and pull your feet in toward your crotch. For a deeper stretch, lean forward.

SIDE-LYING SAVASANA

GREAT FOR:
- End-of-practice relaxation
- End-of-your-rope desperation
- Surprise naps

Savasana, the resting pose that concludes a yoga practice, is usually taken while lying flat on your back in "corpse pose." After your first trimester, this is no longer safe (or comfortable!), but you probably already feel like a corpse, soooo... lay on your left side, to increase blood flow to your baby + placenta as you chill.

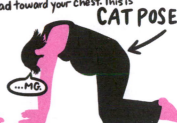

Zzzzz...

PILLOW UNDER HEAD FOR A STR8 SPINE!

BOLSTER OR PILLOW BETWEEN KNEES

normal pregnancies, even in the first trimester! Just let the teacher know before class if you're brand-new to yoga or are very early in your pregnancy, and they'll provide modifications that keep your stretching sesh safe. If the idea of doing yoga right now makes you want to take a nap or barf, listen to your intuition and skip that shit.

TAKE CARE OF YOUR TEETH

Dental health is important during pregnancy because hormones can increase the risk of conditions like gingivitis. Plus, while the miraculous hormone relaxin is loosening up your bod to prepare for birth, it's also going to make your teeth feel a little bit looser in your mouth, which is a creepy feeling! So remember to brush, floss, and visit your dentist, because, you know, you have lots of energy for that! Just don't brush after vomiting, because the stomach acids can scratch the enamel on your teeth.[*] Instead, use mouthwash or smear toothpaste on your teeth with your finger. Yes, you *do* look crazy!

HELP YOUR POOP CHUTE OUT A LITTLE

Your digestion will probably be slow, so eat a little fiber with your dinner, or a whole box of Raisin Bran by the handful after dinner. Fill your grocery cart with "whole foods," if only to create the momentary illusion that you're an earth goddess. Then, when you get home, douse them in salt, sugar, and butter, because *you deserve it! You had a tough day!* Being this mindful of your poop is annoying, but being clogged up with a week's worth of starchy meals is worse; trust us. We bet you've never been more "in tune" with your swelling, noxious body! Yay!

[*] Unless you'd *like* to lose the enamel because your new fuck-the-patriarchy style personal brand is "old crone," which requires dull teeth. In that case, carry on, bad witch.

Eating for Two!

One of the greatest perks of creating a person with your body is that you get to eat extra food to make that person exist. You don't need to eat for two full-grown humans—you actually only need an extra three hundred calories a day—but we know you'll stretch that a little further when your body starts screaming at you for more. Here's what three hundred cals looks like, whether you're going for nutrition or tastiness:

* 1 delicious cup of ice cream

* 10 responsible and overwhelming cups of kale

* 1 middle-of-the-road slice of peanut butter toast

* 1 sneakily eaten Twix in the car

* 37 cucumbers you're "actually weirdly craving"

Warning: Danger Foods!

There are things you're told to never consume while pregnant because you could harm your baby, and, even worse, everyone will judge you for it. Here's the thing: while there are risks associated with the following foods, they are not necessarily death traps.

DELI MEAT AND SOFT CHEESE

If you're craving deli meat and are anxious about food poisoning, you can heat it in the microwave until it's steaming in order to kill bacteria, viruses, or parasites. While deli meat and soft cheese are often the target of listeria suspicions, listeria outbreaks are fairly rare, and recent listeria outbreaks have occurred in frozen vegetables, packaged salads, and bean sprouts. Everybody chill.

SUSHI

Certain types of sushi (shellfish, eel, etc.) are lower than others in mercury, and certain types of sushi are cooked. While there is a risk of parasitic worms in raw fish, many pregnant women have safely eaten it, especially if it's been frozen prior to eating. If you want to lower your risk while still eating sushi, eat it sparingly and at reputable restaurants.

ALCOHOL

The precise effects of controlled substances and medications on a developing fetus are impossible to study because a controlled study would require prescribing potentially dangerous amounts of these substances to pregnant women. If you'd like to partake in a glass of wine here and there, read up and use your best judgment. For some, it's less anxiety-inducing to avoid altogether. If you had a couple of wild nights in the month it took to realize you were pregnant, don't worry. The negative effects of alcohol at that early stage would more likely have resulted in a miscarriage than a birth defect.

COFFEE

Large amounts of caffeine can increase the risk of miscarriage and low birth weight, but those risks are overblown and your morning cup is fiiiiiine—especially if it helps you poop.

TAKE VITAMINS

Pick up a prenatal vitamin that includes DHA. Your body is working hard to make the placenta in the first trimester, so it's pretty easy to get depleted of important vitamins and nutrients. And depleting your body can affect your energy and your mood. Don't worry if you forget a pill or ten—your baby will be fine because your body knows that you no longer matter and has been diverting nutrition to your chia-seed-size kin for several weeks now. If your nausea is so bad that vitamin burps make you yak, consider gummies. A gummy prenatal vitamin is better than a puked-up prenatal vitamin, even if it makes you feel like a giant toddler to take candy medicine.

SEE MORE DOCTORS AND WITCHES

Sure, you don't want to spend your entire pregnancy in a waiting room, but if something is bothering you, now is a great time to "treat yourself" to the miracles of Eastern and/or Western medicine. If it's within your means, see a specialist, acupuncturist, or old woman who shakes a small bag of bird bones at you. Whatever your flavor of care, it'll make you feel good to be nice to your body during this difficult time. If you're having hip or back pain don't wait to seek out a chiropractor,* physical therapist, massage therapist, or spinning babies practitioner. This can decrease the risk of painful complications during pregnancy and labor.

DON'T THROW ALL YOUR MEDS IN THE GARBAGE

If you're taking medications, check in with your provider to find out if there are risks associated with pregnancy. They'll help you decide whether staying on medication is the right decision for you. Since women's bodies are far too boring to study, the effects of many medications on a pregnancy are not fully understood. In these cases, your healthcare provider will weigh the risks to your baby versus the risk of your not taking these meds and offer an informed suggestion for how to proceed. Maybe you should have been born with a penis instead? Boner drugs are very well studied.

Some people may try to scare you off of putting anything but organic veggies into your body during pregnancy, but often, what's good for you is good for your baby. The drugs that make you a stable, functional person who is not constantly full of stress

---

* Look for a chiropractor who is familiar with the Webster technique and isn't afraid of touching a pregnant woman. Then try to relax as she pokes around your round ligament and gives big bear hugs to your pretzeled baby body.

A GUIDE to Forgetting TO TAKE Your *EXPENSIVE* Vitamins!

You spent ninety dollars on these horse pills, and you're supposed to take them every day. Where should you keep them as an easy reminder?

Keep them @ home next to the coffee-maker.

Keep them @ work.

Keep them in your bag for easy access.

Become too nauseous to drink coffee or stomach anything in the morning; forget they are there.

On the subway to work, get so nauseous from smelling other humans that you can't focus on anything at all.

In an effort to hide your pregnancy from suspicious co-workers, put them in the darkest recesses of your desk, where you will never see or think of them.

THIS IS NOT WORKING! YOU NEED TO FIGURE SOMETHING ELSE OUT!!

Set an alarm on your phone.

UM...

Fuck it, this pregnancy is almost OVER.

Alarm never goes off when you're near your phone.

Oh FUCK, you're supposed to keep taking them while you're breastfeeding, too?!

hormones can also be good for the person living within your body. So again—talk to your doctor about the meds you're taking. You may need to make some dosage adjustments or changes to your regimen. Don't go cold turkey without talking to your doctor, and discuss any negative symptoms you're experiencing. You're worth it. Be gentle with yourself.

DON'T DO DRUGS

Most recreational drugs should be strictly avoided during pregnancy, as they pass through the placenta and into your child's system and can harm your child. All that said, America has a long, politically motivated history of demonizing marijuana and categorizing it as a nefarious and harmful substance, and prescribing highly profitable chemical drugs instead. These also pass through the placenta. Just sayin'.

Talk to enough real-ass bitches and you'll find out that many women do use marijuana as medicine during pregnancy, though stigma and fear prevents them from speaking openly about it. During a time when laws and ideas about weed are changing, it's a good idea to do your own research and weigh the medical and legal risks versus the benefits, just like you would with any other medication you ingest during your pregnancy. We aren't telling you it's okay to use marijuana, because it's federally illegal. We're just suggesting that maybe you google "Jamaica Study Marijuana" sometime, if you're interested in this topic.

DRINK! (WATER)

Yeah, we know, right now even water tastes bad somehow. But your blood volume is increasing by 50 percent and that amniotic fluid's gotta come from somewhere, so try to drink some water or seltzer or find a weird pregnant-lady solution like sucking on ice cubes so you look insane and everyone treats you with the caution and care you deserve.

REST THEM WEARY BONES

We know, when someone says, "Sleep now, because this may be your last chance," you want to punch them many times. But really, get some rest. Pregnancy fatigue will come and go, but when it's there, it will hit you like a truck. You'll be feeling more than a little wiped by hormonal changes, the blood you're brewing, and, oh, the fact that you're making a person. Have we mentioned that lately? Pat yourself on your sleepy back. Drop out of unnecessary social events at the last minute. Call out of work from time to time. Rest is a luxury that second-time moms rarely experience, so if this is your first rodeo, don't be a hero! Put your feet up and stare blankly at the ceiling. It's okay. The roller coaster of pregnancy may mean that one day you're surging with energy and on top of the world, and the next you can't keep your peepers open. Give your body what it needs today. Learning to set boundaries with yourself and others is great practice for when you have a baby and quickly learn that "having it all" isn't possible. And stay off your phone, at least sometimes. We know, it's hard for us too.

SHAMELESSLY SELF-CARE

Pregnancy is a rare time when we as women are allowed to take care of ourselves without (as much) guilt. It's odd that it can take having another person in our body for us to realize we can be nice to ourselves, but that's the internalized sexism* that many of us live with. Embrace your newfound free pass to love yourself. Go at your own pace in prenatal yoga class. You can do child's

pose for an hour and no one will judge you. Yoga (and life) was always supposed to be a go-at-your-own-pace thing, but when you're surrounded by a bunch of other sleepy, big-bellied mamas, it's easier to believe it. On your way home from yoga, indulge in whatever makes you feel good: a pedicure, buy a doughnut, sob in the car with no judgment, and ignore work emails. This is your time.

· · · · · · · ·

Remember, at the end of the day, it's about balance. No one expects you to live a sugar-free Gwyneth Paltrow lifestyle. Try to think of healthy choices as less of a punishment and more of a nice thing you are doing for yourself and your baby. So throw some salad in your bacon, buy tubs of Metamucil like your grandma, and take a nap. You've earned it!

· · · · · · · ·

* Internalized sexism is women's involuntary belief in the sexist messages they've received throughout their lives. For example: "I was bad today. I ate cake."

OB-GYNS VERSUS MIDWIVES: WHICH ONE IS JUST THE *WORST*?

Finding the medical care that's right for you and your family will be one of your most important jobs while pregnant. One of the first considerations many will face is the choice of a midwife or ob-gyn (obstetrician-gynecologist). Alarmists will claim that one of these two types of care providers is making it his or her mission to kill you and your baby. But no one is trying to kill you. Both professions include people who range from totally inept to shining examples of humanity. For the most part, they're all trying to keep you and your baby safe. So your preference for one of the two comes down to the kind of care you'd like to receive. Survey your local options to find a provider who feels like a good fit for you. You may find it possible to have the best of both worlds, with an ob-gyn who is willing to be your backup provider to your midwife, in the event that your pregnancy becomes more high-risk.

Pregnancy is long. Very long. Seasons change three times while your baby cooks in your crowded lil' bod, so there's really no reason to rush your decision on a birth plan, though your hormone-addled brain may tell you that everything is a time-sensitive emergency. Searching for the right care provider is a lot like choosing the perfect new pair of winter boots. Did you think we were gonna explain this analogy? We aren't, but you know exactly what we mean.

MIDWIVES VERSUS OB-GYNS— THE ULTIMATE SHOWDOWN

There are many practical differences between the care you receive from an ob-gyn and a midwife, and many similarities too. These considerations aren't always hard rules, but they are some trends we've noted in this chapter.

A Quick Note on Midwives: CNM and CM versus CPM

Certified nurse midwives (CNM) and certified midwives (CM) are crucial and thoroughly educated members of the childbirth community. Both have graduated from an accredited nurse-midwifery master's program and have passed a national exam to earn their professional certifications. They have spent years learning the ins and outs of your ins and outs and are highly qualified to assist you with uncomplicated and complicated births. A CNM or CM can assist you in birthing in a hospital setting, a birth center, at home, or in a fancy hotel if you feel like wrecking someone else's bed instead of your own.

The credentials for those who identify themselves as a CPM (certified professional midwife) are quite different. Legal in only twenty-eight states and sometimes operating outside of the law, a CPM can become a "certified midwife" through an online course and an apprenticeship with an existing CPM. They are not recognized as midwives by the Accreditation Commission for Midwifery Education and have not been required to pass the national exam.

Birth is complicated and often unpredictable, so choosing a well-trained and trusted care provider is crucial to your birth experience and to the health of yourself and your child, no matter what kind of birth you want to have. When interviewing prospective midwives, always come prepared with questions about credentials and experience so you can make the most informed decision for your family.

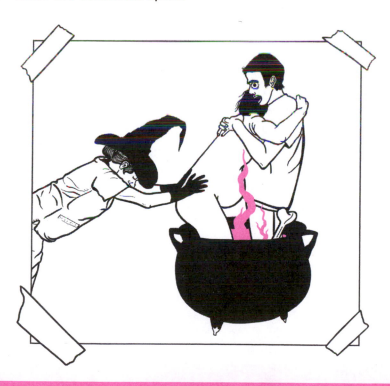

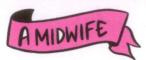

A MIDWIFE

- Has a graduate degree (assuming CNM or CM—see sidebar: "A Quick Note on Midwives: CNM and CM versus CPM").
- Said degree is very specialized to the care of a pregnant woman.
- Will never try to cut you open. But can refer you to a doctor who can, if necessary.
- Incredibly unlikely to be a man.
- Depending on the midwife and the state you reside in, she can sometimes perform home births, sometimes deliver at a birth center or hospital, and sometimes both.
- More hands-off when it comes to optional testing and procedures than an MD.
- More hands-on when it comes to checking in with your mental health, helping you prepare your life for the changes a baby brings, and is more likely to talk to you about your feelings.
- More likely to prescribe holistic remedies, such as acupuncture.
- Around while you labor, and generally more knowledgeable than OBs on laboring positions that may help move your baby down, creating a shorter and easier labor.
- Usually provides more postpartum care and check-ins.
- Some provide circumcisions, if desired by the parent.

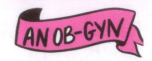

AN OB-GYN

- Has a big fancy degree that took a lot of time.
- Said degree involved studying a lot of things that are not always 100 percent relevant to your care.
- Knows how to cut you open, which is quite useful when you need to be cut open.
- About 50 percent chance of being a man.
- Almost always delivers in a hospital.
- Statistically more likely to use interventions during labor, such as labor-induction medications like Pitocin and Cervidil, episiotomy procedures, forceps, and C-sections.

Authors Note: Interventions are sometimes medically necessary, and thank goodness they are available.

- May be more rigorous in their use of blood tests and screenings, if you're worried about hereditary illness or birth defects.
- Can perform circumcisions, if desired by the parent.
- Unless there are complications, will not be around much during your labor until you are ready to deliver.

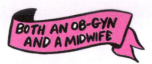

BOTH AN OB-GYN AND A MIDWIFE

- Can provide prenatal care for normal and high-risk pregnancies. (If you are high-risk, you can see both.)

- Can order tests to monitor your and your baby's health, including ultrasounds and blood work.

- Can write prescriptions and provide referrals to physical, chiropractic, and other complementary therapies, which can really help in both the prenatal and postpartum periods.

- Can assist you in attempting an unmedicated birth, if that's your plan. You'll notice that we didn't say "natural," because all birth is natural, unless you are a pregnant cyborg, or Arnold Schwarzenegger in that fever dream of a nineties' feature film *Junior.*

- Can be fired at any time by you. If you are unhappy with the care you are receiving, you should absolutely find someone who does it better. You deserve it.

- Wants to help you safely deliver a healthy baby.

DID YOU FRIGGIN' KNOW?

An **episiotomy** is an incision made into the perineum (the area between vag and butt) in order to more quickly facilitate birth. Episiotomy rates have dropped drastically over the past couple of decades, as evidence suggests it is rarely medically necessary or beneficial. Episiotomies can lead to serious pain, injury, or increased recovery times compared to spontaneous tears (when your perineum tears on its own as you're pushing the baby out). If concerned, ask your doctor how often they perform this procedure. Episiotomies: 'taint necessary.

CONSIDERATIONS FOR ANY PROVIDER

Is it a group practice? How many people will you be showing your vag to?

Unless your ob-gyn is a small-town, old-timey, no-nonsense movie character doctor whose office is behind the general store, *most* midwives and doctors operate under the umbrella of a group practice. This is so they can all go in on utilities and the internet bill and still have pizza money left over at the end of the week. If you choose a provider from a shared practice, you may see a different person at each of your visits, and any of them might be the one to deliver your baby. Try your best to schedule checkups with each of these providers so they all get a chance to see your vagina and you make sure you're comfortable and feel respected by all of them. Don't be afraid to speak up for yourself—if one member of the practice is off-putting, the rest want to hear about it.

Are you happy with your provider and comfortable while showing your vag to them?

Maybe you want someone who spends a lot of time listening to your concerns, or maybe you prefer someone who cuts to the chase. Remember, whether they are an ob-gyn or a midwife, this person's demeanor will likely remain similar when you are in labor. Al-though, again, there is always the chance that you'll go into labor on a day when your chosen provider is not on call and then none of this matters! The unpredictability of labor is unfortunately something you should get used to, but that doesn't mean you aren't allowed to have high standards for the way you are treated.

Are you high-risk?

Your care provider may make an assessment early on that you are high-risk, but it can happen at any point in your pregnancy and can impact your choice of providers and alter your birth plan. A high-risk pregnancy is still most often a healthy one, so don't freak out too much; people's bodies are complicated, and everyone responds to pregnancy differently. Being classified as high-risk simply means that your provider will watch you and your baby more closely during pregnancy and will probably require you to birth at a hospital. You may be considered high-risk if you:

- are "advanced maternal age" (AMA), which means that you have two or more wrinkles on your face.
- are younger than seventeen.
- are significantly overweight.
- are pregnant with more than one baby, bless your crowded heart.
- have a chronic disease.

- develop gestational diabetes, which you'll be tested for at twenty weeks.
- develop preeclampsia, a rare complication that raises blood pressure and causes sudden and dramatic swelling. For more on preeclampsia, see "Weird Symptoms that Mean You Should Call Your Doctor/Midwife," page 64.
- are taking certain medications that require close monitoring.

If you've been classified as high-risk, remember: high risk equals high reward. That's from stock market stuff, but it means you're gonna be rich!

Where do you want to spit out this baby?

While one of the writers of this book gave birth in a Honda Fit, American women by and large choose one of three places to birth: a hospital, a birthing center, or at home.

Hospitals are a great choice for high-risk pregnancies; if you know you'll want narcotic pain relief, an epidural, or nitrous gas; or if having a medical team behind you makes you feel safe. Birthing centers are, in general, nicer places to labor because they provide the freedom typical of midwifery care with quick access to a hospital if it were to become necessary, and they are likely to have birthing tubs with spa jets so you can live your best labor life. Unfortunately, birthing centers are uncommon in many parts of the country. At a hospital, you may be required to wear a fetal monitor, and this may mean staying on your back in bed. Birthing centers typically do intermittent fetal monitoring, allowing you the freedom to take advantage of their jetted bathtubs and showers for pain relief and relaxation. Women who feel safest in their own private space may opt to birth at home with a midwife, but we'll talk about this more in "Home Birth: So You've Decided to Shit in a Pool," page 88.

. . . .

Wherever you choose to bleed, make sure that you create a plan with your birthing partner or doula for how everyone will get there when the time comes. You will not feel like coordinating a team of people while your cervix is dilating to the size of an authentic Brooklyn bagel.

WEIRD THINGS THAT HAPPEN TO YOU AT THE DOCTOR NOW THAT YOU'RE PREGNANT

Before pregnancy, your provider probs did a quick swab down there and you got birth control for days, but now it's a different story.

YOU PEE INTO CUPS NEARLY CONSTANTLY

Suddenly everyone loves to look at your pee! Get used to handing it to a surprisingly cheerful nurse* who handles other people's blood and pee all day. She's looking for signs of gestational diabetes, infection, or protein in your urine, which can be a sign of pre-eclampsia.

BUTT SWABS, OH BOY!

You thought prying open your vagina with a speculum was awkward. Now people are sticking a big Q-tip into your butthole to test for Group B strep. Intimate!

QUESTIONS, SO MANY QUESTIONS

What the heck are you doing with yourself? Inquiring minds want to know. Share what you can, even if you're somewhat ashamed of your habits, so that your doctor can help advise you on how to improve them. If your doctor is overly judgmental, we sympathize. Maybe you *do* eat a little too much fish. We get it.

NEW PEOPLE LOOKING AT YOUR VAGINA ALL THE TIME

In a group practice, you won't always see the same doctor, and as the frequency of visits increases later in your pregnancy, it will feel like your vagina is speed-dating in hopes of marrying a nice doctor. Good luck, little lady!

* It's easy to bitch about the grumpy nurses, but how do the nice ones stay sooo nice?!

Sonograms: Finding Out if Your Baby Is Photogenic

At some point in your pregnancy, your ob-gyn or midwife will likely want you to have a sonogram. Sonograms are done for many reasons, generally to check up on the size and health of the developing fetus, but it's hard not to focus on the *real* reason for sonograms—finding out how photogenic your baby is!

A CUTE BABY AT FOUR WEEKS

At this stage you may not even be 100 percent sure you're pregnant, so the pic is all about your baby making herself known.

A CUTE BABY AT TWELVE WEEKS

At twelve weeks, your baby's looking pretty skeletal, so getting a good pic is all about finding his or her angles. The head-on pics look notoriously skull-like, so try to get them to snap something from the side.

A CUTE BABY AT THIRTY-THREE WEEKS

Many moms won't even get a sonogram this late in the game, but if you can find a medical excuse to swing it, this is the true glamour shot of fetal documentation. Your baby's cheeks are filling out, and they are looking full-human. The trick is getting the baby to hold still and not put a hand in front of their face—an amateur fetal move.

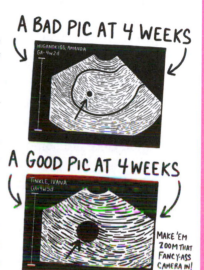

A BAD PIC AT 4 WEEKS

HUGANOKISS, AMANDA
GA·4w2d

A GOOD PIC AT 4 WEEKS

TINKLE, IVANA
GA·4w5d

MAKE 'EM ZOOM THAT FANCY-ASS CAMERA IN!

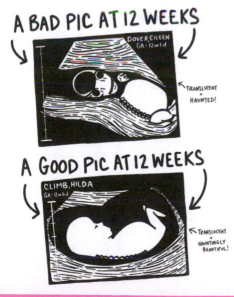

A BAD PIC AT 12 WEEKS

DOVER, EILEEN
GA·12w1d

TRANSLUCENT + HAUNTED!

A GOOD PIC AT 12 WEEKS

CLIMB, HILDA
GA·12w6d

TRANSLUCENT + HAUNTINGLY BEAUTIFUL!

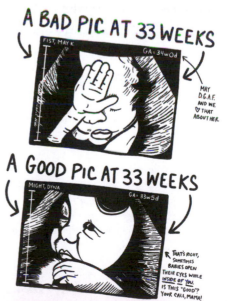

A BAD PIC AT 33 WEEKS

FIST, MAY K
GA=34w0d

MAY D.G.A.F. AND WE ♡ THAT ABOUT HER.

A GOOD PIC AT 33 WEEKS

MIGHT, DYNA
GA=33w5d

THAT'S RIGHT, SOMETIMES BABIES OPEN THEIR EYES WHILE INSIDE OF YOU. IS THIS "GOOD"? YOUR CALL, MAMA!

SOMEBODY HELP ME! THERE'S A BABY IN MY BODY!

In addition to seeking out health professionals, you and your partner may want to get some hands-on knowledge of what's in store, especially if you haven't spent a lot of time around babies or women in labor. Here are some things you might want to do to prepare.

SIGN UP FOR CHILDBIRTH CLASSES

There are many different styles of childbirth classes, but they all pretty much have the same goal: to help you cope with the fact that the human inside of your body has to come out soon. Learning the stages of labor and delivery helps build your confidence as you approach the big day. Classes are also an opportunity to meet other expectant moms in your 'hood. Nothing helps a friendship grow faster than simulating labor growls together while a teacher holds up giant illustrations of dilated cervixes!*

If you're planning to give birth in a hospital, ask them about their class offerings. This is a good way to tour the facility and get to know their rules and regulations while you learn some useful birthing techniques. Want more options? Do a search for childbirth education in your area: Lamaze, Bradley method, Alexander technique, and hypnobirthing† are all very popular and very different methods of preparation.

TAKE TO THE INTERNET, IF YOU'RE SOCIALLY AWKWARD

If a group class is not your scene, there are tons of resources online to help you prepare for whatever sort of birth you're aiming to have. From free YouTube videos to extensive PDF e-books on how to identify the shape of your own pelvic bones, there are plenty of tools to help you understand the ways in which your body is about to explode and how to help it do so more easily.

---

* Seriously, grab the phone numbers for some of these women so you can text them "WTF?!" in a few months when you're both dealing with newborns.

† Hard-core "hypnomoms" claim that the technique is so powerful that some women actually achieve "orgasmic births." Though everything in our rational minds tells us that this is nearly impossible, we prefer to cling desperately to the idea that there are some women getting off while giving birth; *GET IT!*

FIND A BABY-CARE CLASS

These classes can be helpful, especially if you don't have a ton of experience with newborns. They'll usually teach you some breastfeeding techniques, tips for newborn health, ways to soothe your baby; demystify puzzling baby carriers; help hone your swaddle game; and let you hold a floppy, scuffed-up old baby doll and imagine it's your own baby for a little bit. Don't worry about dropping the doll on its head; there's a reason it's already scuffed. If your class offers infant CPR, great! If not, it's a good idea to take one of those too. Babies choke a lot, and knowing what to do is important; not just for safety but also to avoid spinning in a shame and regret spiral every time they cough.

HOLD YOUR FRIEND'S BABY FOR A FEW MINUTES

She needs a break anyway, so point her tired ass toward bed and snuggle up in a rocking chair with that baby to get some sweet cuddles in. Sniff that baby head, do that weird thing women do where we closely examine a baby's hands like there are tiny instructions written on them, and cry a little if you need to. We won't tell. If you're far enough along,

your boobs might start tingling and leaking when the baby cries, and that's a weird thing you might as well get used to now!

NETFLIX AND CHILL

Check out a birth documentary or *Call the Midwife* or something. Honestly, just watch everything you can; you are getting fatter by the moment and the TV is your friend. Just try to avoid movies about unwanted pregnancies and reluctant dads, because those will not scratch the right itch right now!

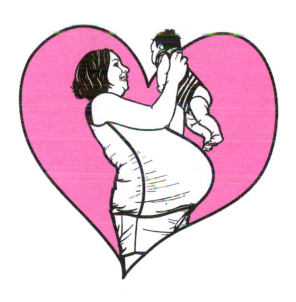

Things to Force Your Partner/Birth Team to Read

There's an old saying: a woman becomes a mother when she finds out she's pregnant, and a man becomes a father when he meets his baby. This is extremely manipulative, because the first half of the quote has you like, "Aww, so true, I *do* already feel like a mother," and the second half basically enables men to pretend like nothing is happening until your vagina coughs out a tiny squirming human who looks like them. Let's fuck with this status quo, shall we?

During pregnancy, women tend to hungrily consume information on pregnancy, birth, and child-rearing, while their partners tend to . . . not do that. This, like most emotional labor that we perform, is unfair bullshit. So we've done the emotional labor of preparing a list of required reading for partners, because at least *we* are getting paid. In hetero couples, fathers are half the parenting team and should be as prepared as mothers as they enter this new stage of life. You might as well go ahead and read these too, so you can cite them like a scholarly bitch when people claim you're doing something wrong.

A BOOK THAT LINES UP WITH YOUR BIRTH PLAN

If you're planning an unmedicated or home birth, *Ina May's Guide to Childbirth* is widely considered to be the bible, but there are great books for every kind of birthing experience, from a planned C-section to a VBAC. Whatever your plan, your loved ones can best assist you in implementing it if they have a thorough and nuanced understanding of what to expect, what the challenges may be, and what recovery looks like.

A TERRIBLY TOXIC MOMMY MESSAGE BOARD

Have your partner read this so they understand what it's like to be a new mother in the world and how important it is to check sources when googling baby stuff. This may not seem important now, but at 3:00 a.m. when your kid won't sleep and your husband mansplains some crazy shit he read on BabyCenter, you'll wish you had told him to ignore BabyCenter.

A BOOK THAT WILL KEEP YOUR PARTNER FROM FREAKING OUT DURING YOUR LABOR

We recommend that all nonprofessionals who are attending your birth read the book *The Birth Partner: A Complete Guide to Childbirth for Dads, Doulas, and Other Labor Companions* by Penny Simkin. It's a great primer on the actual process of birth that covers a lot of pretty scientific info in a digestible form, empowering your chosen birth team to be educated, helpful, and compassionate.

BONUS BOOK: FOR ANYONE WHO SIDE-EYES YOU WHEN YOU EAT SUSHI OR DRINK A BEER

Gift them a copy of *Expecting Better: Why the Conventional Pregnancy Wisdom Is Wrong—and What You Really Need to Know* by Emily Oster. This well-researched book debunks a lot of traditional pregnancy wisdom with modern science, and, more important, it treats pregnant women like intelligent human beings capable of making their own decisions about their health and the health of their baby.

THIS BOOK

Obviously. Please buy everyone you know a copy; we have children to feed.

WEIRD SECOND-TRIMESTER PREGNANCY SYMPTOMS

As your pregnancy progresses into the second trimester, you may feel a little less nauseous and a little more like there's a life inside you. And yet, the functions of your body will continue to be . . . weird. Here are some strange symptoms you may experience midpregnancy.

YOUR BABY SEEMS TO BE TRAINING FOR THE OLYMPICS

In the second trimester, you'll probably start to feel the baby move. In your first pregnancy, it may take longer to recognize those strange little baby kicks, which often feel like gas bubbles. Historically, feeling the baby move inside you is called "quickening," which sounds very magical, like you're conjuring a little person. Honestly, you are! In your eagerness for your partner to feel those kicks, you may find yourself stuffing his or her hand into the top of your stretchy waistband like a horny teen. And much like horny teens, it may take some time for this experience to be mutually satisfying. But make no mistake, soon you'll both be feeling it.

At some point in the second trimester, your baby will become much stronger. You know that feeling when you're swimming in a body of water and you feel something big brush up against your leg, and it was *definitely* alive and you have no idea what it was? Yeah, it's a lot like that. Magical, right?

YOU'VE GOT THE HICCUPS . . . IN YOUR BUTT?

You might feel your baby hiccup inside you and wonder what she's been drinking. The answer: amniotic fluid. Apparently she needs to learn to hold hers. In the meantime, she'll be thumping that bass beat, which you may even feel in your vagina or butt. Ah, the miracle of life!

YOU DON'T WANT TO BARF EVERYTHING!

In the second trimester, many women find their nausea starts to subside and they have renewed energy. If this is you, take advantage of it while you can, because in late pregnancy you may tire of hauling yourself around. Get out of the house while you can, even if it's just to drive to the baby store, stare at overpriced onesies, burst into tears, buy only a bar of chocolate, and go home.

So what is going on with your body, exactly?

During pregnancy, your **uterus**, a normally normal-size organ, expands to house a huge human baby. Within the uterus, the **placenta** is also formed via fetal and maternal cells. This is basically where you and your baby merge. The placenta connects the baby to the uterine wall via the **umbilical cord**, supplying nutrients to your baby and allowing your baby to remove their waste into you (in effect they're kind of shitting into your bloodstream, another neat metaphor for motherhood).

Between conception and birth, your uterus expands to be five hundred times larger. Everything else in your tummy gets shoved up and to the sides. Your joints will loosen, and your hip bones will move to make way for your baby's birth. Your spine will also become more curved in order to accommodate the weight of your belly so that you're not falling over all the time. As early as six weeks into pregnancy your **boobs** will get bigger (a blessing or curse depending on how you look at it). As blood flows to expand the glandular tissue that produces milk, the veins on your breasts may become more visible and your **areolas** will darken and increase in size.

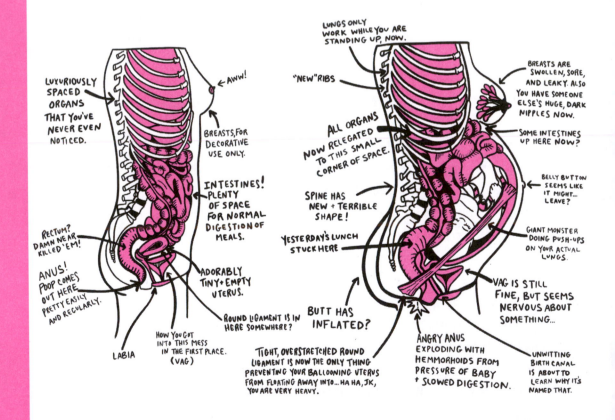

LUXURIOUSLY SPACED ORGANS THAT YOU'VE NEVER EVEN NOTICED.

←AWW!

BREASTS, FOR DECORATIVE USE ONLY.

INTESTINES! PLENTY OF SPACE FOR NORMAL DIGESTION OF MEALS.

RECTUM? DAMN NEAR KILLED 'EM!

ANUS! POOP COMES OUT HERE PRETTY EASILY AND REGULARLY.

ADORABLY TINY + EMPTY UTERUS.

ROUND LIGAMENT IS IN HERE SOMEWHERE?

LABIA

HOW YOU GOT INTO THIS MESS IN THE FIRST PLACE. (VAG)

LUNGS ONLY WORK WHILE YOU ARE STANDING UP, NOW.

"NEW" RIBS

ALL ORGANS NOW RELEGATED TO THIS SMALL CORNER OF SPACE.

SPINE HAS NEW + TERRIBLE SHAPE!

YESTERDAY'S LUNCH STUCK HERE

BUTT HAS INFLATED?

BREASTS ARE SWOLLEN, SORE, AND LEAKY. ALSO YOU HAVE SOMEONE ELSE'S HUGE, DARK NIPPLES NOW.

SOME INTESTINES UP HERE NOW?

BELLY BUTTON SEEMS LIKE IT MIGHT... LEAVE?

GIANT MONSTER DOING PUSH-UPS ON YOUR ACTUAL LUNGS.

VAG IS STILL FINE, BUT SEEMS NERVOUS ABOUT SOMETHING...

TIGHT, OVERSTRETCHED ROUND LIGAMENT IS NOW THE ONLY THING PREVENTING YOUR BALLOONING UTERUS FROM FLOATING AWAY INTO... HA HA, JK, YOU ARE VERY HEAVY.

ANGRY ANUS EXPLODING WITH HEMMORHOIDS FROM PRESSURE OF BABY + SLOWED DIGESTION.

UNWITTING BIRTH CANAL IS ABOUT TO LEARN WHY IT'S NAMED THAT.

As your uterus inflates like a balloon, it is held in place by two **round ligaments** that connect to your pelvis/groin almost like the ropes keeping the balloons from floating away in a Thanksgiving Day parade.

Unfortunately, ligaments are made of fibrous connective tissue and are not very stretchy. This means that as your uterus grows, they tend to get very tight, which can cause round ligament pain, especially if the alignment of your hips is off. Since ligaments stretch and contract very slowly, this pain tends to be triggered by fast movements, such as sneezing or coughing, rolling over in bed, standing up quickly, or really trying to do anything at a faster-than-your-nana pace.

You can ease this pain by practicing good balance and posture, seeing a chiropractor or physical therapist, wearing a belly-support belt,[*] doing the gentle yoga stretches on page 19, or by massaging the area where the round ligament meets your hip.

* * * * * * * * * *
* For more on belly support, see "Ugh, Maternity 'Fashion,'" page 51.

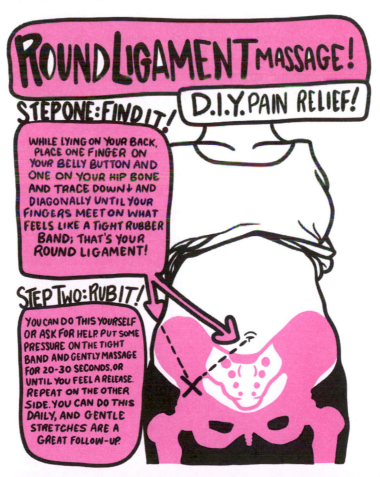

If your energy does not return, or your nausea does not subside, congrats! You're having a tough pregnancy. Unfortunately, this is a very normal possibility, but there are some advantages too. Milk the sympathy while you can and make outrageous demands of your loved ones.

YOU WANT ALL THE SIDES, ALL THE TOPPINGS

If your nausea is finally dissipating, have at it, lady! Though you don't necessarily need to make up for lost time. Your baby is still pretty small and needs minimal calories. There will be *plenty* of time for gorging yourself in the third trimester, when you're big and tired and have few other coping mechanisms to soothe your sensitive hormonal self. But please, enjoy food now that you can.

YOUR STOMACH IS ON FIRE

Pregnancy hormones relax the valve between your stomach and esophagus, which means you may suffer from heartburn or turn into a full-blown dragon. Eat smaller, more frequent meals, avoid problem foods, and don't lie down after eating (we know, shouldn't you be entitled to these things now?!). Antacids such as TUMS should be safe, but avoid anything containing sodium bicarbonate, such as Rolaids or Alka-Seltzer. Some people find papaya enzyme tablets to be helpful, too.

YOU SEEM HIGH

If you haven't already been hit by pregnancy exhaustion and brain fog, you may start to have days where you're just kind of like, "Huh?" You'll walk in a daze, half processing information, forgetting your phone is in your hand, and forgetting your hand is attached to your body. This is great preparation for those first few months* when your child's incessant demands zap your brainpower.

YOU'RE HORNY AF

With the renewed energy of the second trimester and all the extra fluid and hormones coursing through you, you might be DTFAF!† Your body is producing more estrogen in a single day than a nonpregnant woman's ovaries do in three years! Take that, skinny bitches! If you're feeling frisky, enjoy it while you still can. You might find your arousal dissipates in the third trimester, not to mention you may have a harder time maneuvering during sex and solo play. Get it, EMELTF!‡

* . . . years
† Down to Fuck As Fuck
‡ Expecting Mom Enjoying Loving to Fuck

YOU'RE BREATHING LIKE A TODDLER ON A TRAMPOLINE

You may find yourself out of breath from simple activities as your body tries to circulate all that new blood. Plus, as your uterus grows, it starts to squish other organs out of the way, crowding your little lungs. You'd think the human body could've evolved something better than just smushing everything into the same space, but it didn't, and here we are, huffing and puffing up the stairs.

YOU'RE DREAMIN'!

Many women report more vivid and frequent dreams during pregnancy. If yours are bad, try to find ways to unwind before bed, like reading or sex or watching Mark Ruffalo movies. Then maybe instead of bad dreams about how the baby arrived and you forgot to buy a crib, you'll have sexy dreams about Mark Ruffalo building you a you-size fuck crib.

YOUR BELLY IS ITCHY AND TIGHT AND EVERYTHING IS THE WORST

Stretching skin and hormonal changes may make you very itchy, and this can be pretty unbearable. Treat your belly like a beached whale that needs to be kept cool and wet, and incessantly dump on buckets of lotion until help arrives. Do you have one of those hammocks that they use to transfer whales? Yeah, get in that thing and lube up.

YOUR SKIN IS CHANGING

Some women develop a harmless but confusing dark line going down the center of their abdomen, called a **linea nigra**. It's caused by an increase in the hormones that help you produce melanin, which means you may also suffer from **melasma** (darkened patches of skin on the face) or **darkened nipples**. Honestly, we think you pull it off really well. If you're prone to sunburn, take heed: your skin is more sensitive while pregnant, and burning an achy, tight belly is *the worst,* so lather up with SPF 50 and reapply often. If you're prone to freckles, you may get more. *A lot* more, sometimes. This is also due to an increase in melanin. Lighter freckles may get darker. Consider connecting them to form constellations and repeat the following mantra: *I am the entire universe. Fear me.*

YOUR PELVIS IS WOBBLY

For years it held you up so easily, and now you're feeling like an overstretched Slinky stuffed into a romper. Your body is producing the hormone relaxin (not to be confused with relaxin', which is way more fun), so your ligaments, muscles, joints, and everything you rely on to stand upright are loosening to prepare for labor. If your wobble is

Nesting: An Excuse to Incur Debt

Once the exhaustion of the first trimester fades, your creepy animal brain switches to the next task at hand: building your nest. What's your favorite bird? Yeah, you're like a fat one of those! When the nesting instinct kicks in hard, you may find yourself scrubbing the inside of drawers you've literally never opened before and organizing your books by color because you saw it on Pinterest. Be careful about spending big money on things like furniture, or you might end up with a *very* deep, light-colored couch called "the Lounger" that seemed like a good decision when you were pregnant and needed everything to be a bed. Six months later, when it is covered in stains and impossible to stand up from while holding a sleeping baby, your weird hormones will make you feel incredibly guilty about the debt you've incurred at Crate & Barrel, and you'll want to set the thing on fire at least twice a day. Hypothetically speaking.

Now's a great time to prepare your living space for the baby and create systems that will make it easier to manage life when you're too tired to speak in full sentences. Have a male partner who doesn't understand how to do anything around the house, because his mom did it all? Fuuuuck that shit; get a label maker. Men are sometimes too proud to ask for help and sometimes so helpless they ask for help before they've made any attempt at doing a thing in the first place. Luckily they seem to be pretty good at following direct orders. A label maker allows you to boss him around while you're not even in the room and makes your organizational efforts transparent and easy to follow, so when he ignores the labels you can say things like "It's literally written right there!"

Once the baby arrives, you will need to have very good delegation skills, so start flexing that muscle now. Sure, you could do the laundry, but your partner needs to get used to helping. Ideally, you shouldn't have to ask a grown man to do laundry, or throw away those wet pieces of paper from between pieces of prosciutto that he leaves all over the kitchen counter like receipts he intends to file, but it's going to take a lot of baby steps on both sides to erase the long-standing tradition of men being helpless babies whom we must take care of even when our body is a literal open wound. Bottom line: you can't do everything, and the sooner you both learn that, the happier you'll be.

SET UP YOUR MOM STATION

Nesting isn't just for baby prep; you're also preparing for your own shift into motherhood. For the first few weeks after your birth, you'll be spending a lot of time in bed with a sleepy, cute, needy, and charmingly boring person. Think of this as a "staycation," but one where you get paler and more sleep-deprived the longer you're there.

As you nest, make some space in your nightstand by moving all vibrators to the closet* since you will likely not want anything vibrating near your vagina for many weeks. In their place, we recommend: headphones

---

* Now is a good time to decide on a secure place to store any sex toys you may not want your soon-to-be-mobile-and-very-curious toddler to find. This may not seem important now, but you'll wish you listened when your darling child enters the kitchen singing "Twinkle Twinkle Little Star" into your vibrator like it's a microphone and you want to be swallowed up by the earth.

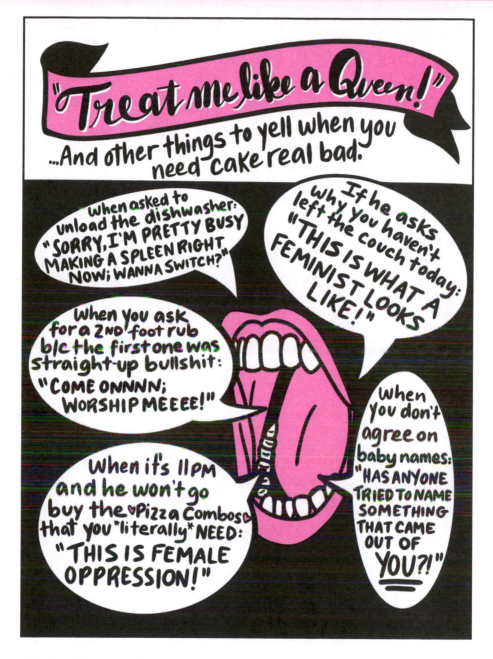

and a tablet for binge-watching, extra-long charging cables, dry shampoo for your greasy-ass third-day hair, hair ties, sore-boob supplies, sore-vagina supplies, pain meds, water bottles or water pitcher, extra onesies, lip balm, and, obviously, this book. Your future, extremely zonked mess-of-a-perfect-mom-self thanks you.

My friend said she "loved every moment of being pregnant"— is it okay to murder her?

While it is not legally or morally okay to end another person's life, we're with you, boo. When your mouth tastes like puke and you're getting shooting pains inside of your vagina (literally called "lightning crotch"* by the professional medical community), the last thing you want to hear is how easy it was for someone else.

It's common to internalize these feelings and wonder if there's something wrong with you. Nope. Your mildly obnoxious friend is probably lying, exaggerating, or suffering from mom brain. Summon all of your compassion and nod your head politely, then send a snarky text about it to someone who gets you.

. . . .
* We did not make this one up.

getting in the way of your life, you might try prenatal physical therapy, a support belt, or duct tape in a pinch.

NONE OF THE ABOVE

One of the weirdest things about pregnancy is that yours is totally unique, so if you're missing out on many of the symptoms we've mentioned, consider yourself lucky. Maybe double-check to see if you actually are pregnant, but if you are and you're still just a happy, healthy, cheerful woman, congrats— we hate you! But seriously, it's okay to be excited about becoming a mom and taking this all in stride. We're just projecting some feelings right now, okay?

LOVE THAT BUMP, GIRL

In media, we generally see the same version of pregnant women—rail-thin with a big belly. Their faces and ankles aren't bloated because they aren't actually pregnant—they're actresses and models wearing prosthetics. Most of us won't look like these women in real life, nor should we be expected to. While unrealistic expectations make many of us preggo ladies feel like we're too much or not enough, we're all beautiful goddesses of varying lumpy shapes. Here's what that might look like for you.

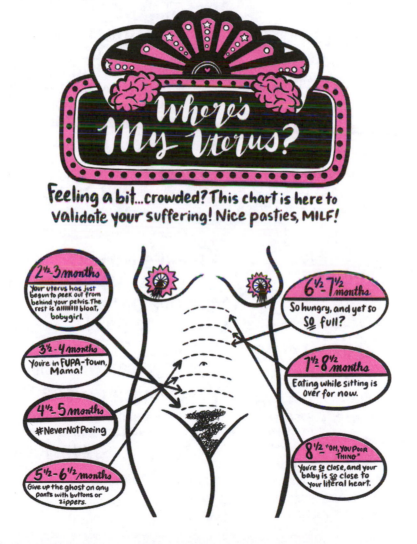

Where's My Uterus?

Feeling a bit...crowded? This chart is here to validate your suffering! Nice pasties, MILF!

2½–3 months — Your uterus has just begun to peek out from behind your pelvis. The rest is allllllll bloat, babygirl.

3½–4 months — You're in FUPA-town, Mama!

4½–5 months — #NeverNotPeeing

5½–6½ months — Give up the ghost on any pants with buttons or zippers.

6½–7½ months — So hungry, and yet so SO full?

7½–8½ months — Eating while sitting is over for now.

8½ "OH, YOU POOR THING" — You're so close, and your baby is so close to your literal heart.

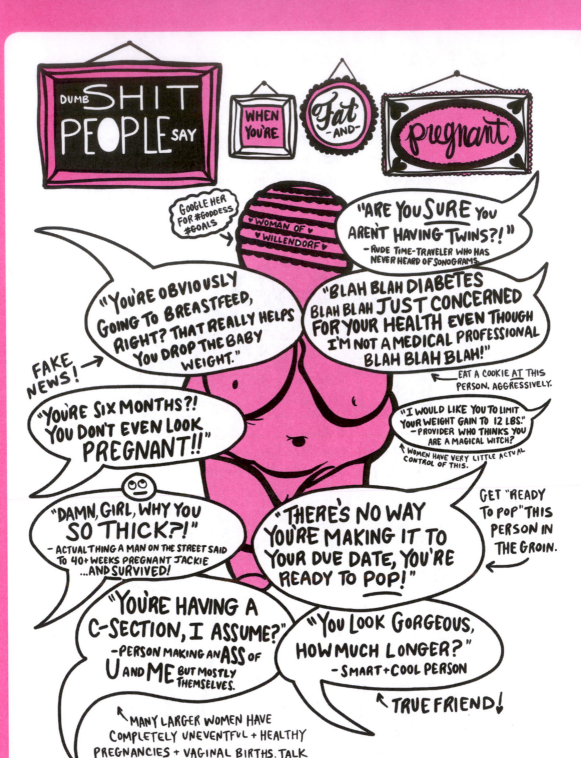

Your Body as Public Property

Once visibly pregnant, you'll receive lots of "fun" comments from friends, family, and strangers. People feel compelled to weigh in on women's bodies, especially now that you're two people in one. You have a right to be annoyed by unnecessary questions, advice, or bizarre characterizations of what the size and shape of your body "means" to them. Remember that people are dumb and their rude comments bear no reflection on you, your health, or your worth.

COMMENTS ABOUT YOUR WEIGHT AND UNSOLICITED WEIGHT-LOSS ADVICE

If, like many women, your weight skyrockets during pregnancy, you'll probably get some comments on how to rein it in. Ugh, sorry. If, like many women, you were born with a small frame, you'll probably get comments about needing to gain more weight. Ugh, sorry. A nice "I'm trying to stay more body-positive than that; I feel really healthy right now" can really throw a hater off their game. For every woman who is fat-shamed during her pregnancy, there's a woman who is told she's not gaining enough weight and should be less vain. For every woman told that she's too "overweight" to deliver vaginally, another woman is told her body is too small to deliver the baby she grew inside of it.

LOVING LOOKS FROM STRANGERS

Even positive attention can sometimes feel terrible. Strangers will stop you on the street to say congratulations or reach out and touch your belly like it's a ripe melon they're considering at the market. They mean well, but as a tired pregnant woman, you don't always want to stop and explain your body. Offering a curt "Thanks but it's really none of your business" is fine by us.

CATCALLS?

Don't be surprised if you find yourself getting checked out or catcalled while pregnant. Some men view your visible ability to reproduce as a sign that you are always down for D, even while fully fertilized. You are more than welcome to scream at anyone who offers up unwelcome overtures (assuming you feel safe doing so).

Women can't seem to have a body without being judged for it, so let's all try to support one another, rather than supporting the patriarchal ideas forced on us by dumb, old white dudes who can't make babies in their bodies. You're great. Haters. Are. Just. Jealous.

PRE-BUMP FATNESS

Media rarely represents the awkward pre-bump phase, where your belly is just a little bit fatter than before. "Hmm, you don't really look pregnant," people might say. And while you know you're perfectly healthy and normal, you might fear the prospect of people wondering if you've put on a few pounds (as if weight gain were a crime on par with murder). This is one of the many ways pregnancy makes us feel like an awkward teenager going through puberty. You can either hide your lil' belly under large shirts or "show it off" with tighter clothes. Do what feels comfortable, and ignore what your grandmother has to say about the red tents pregnant women were banished to in her day. You're forging the way for the next generation of pregnant women and every "F you" you send the patriarchy is a tiny step forward for all of us. Also, Grandma might not be the most realistic touchstone for modern-day motherhood. She's a little nuts, you know?

THE EARLY-BIRD BUMP BUFFET

On the other hand, you might look pregnant the moment you take a positive pregnancy test. You're in the unenviable position of having strangers asking you about your pregnancy for nine straight months. Rude people will say things like "Any day now, huh?" or "Are you sure it's not twins?" Even healthcare providers will offend with their "helpful" suggestions about the rate at which you're gaining weight, as if you'd made it your goal to be enormous. It's okay! Pregnant women expand.

MY BABY TOO BOOTYLICIOUS FOR YA

Some women "carry their baby in their ass," which is a horribly offensive and biologically inaccurate way of describing the normal widening of hips and weight gain in your booty. If you've never had a butt before, enjoy it! It, like most pregnancy changes, is temporary.

· · · · · · · ·

Whether you're a grower or a shower, it's important to remember that none of us has it easy. Try not to direct your rage at the other women who seem to have it "better." The real enemy is the expectation that our bodies should be any one way in the first place. We're all unique—why should our pregnancies be any different?

MAKING YOUR PREGNANCY KNOWN

> You don't have to "announce" your pregnancy. It's totally fine to leave it at "Hey, I'm pregnant." Here are some possible considerations when letting people know what's up.

REVEALING THE DUE DATE

This is one of the first things people will want to know. Coworkers will want to start planning for your absence. Family may want to start making plans to descend on you.

SHARING PHOTOS

If you feel like sharing, many loved ones will enjoy photographic evidence of your pregnancy. You don't *have* to share pics of yourself or your sonograms, but it could mean a lot to family and friends who can't see you in person. If you're sharing on social media, make sure to set your privacy settings appropriately, because Aunt Candy hits share on every damn thing she sees, and maybe you don't want Aunt Candy's friends from her Silver Singles Cruise making weird comments about your belly.

DEALING WITH PEOPLE WHO ARE NOSY ABOUT YOUR BIRTH PLAN

Sometimes people will just walk right up and ask what "kind" of a birth you're having. It's weird and rude, but it happens. Legit and valid answers include "One where a baby is born," and "Hmm, probably a moon birth, but not totally sure yet because of the whole gravity situation." If you're down to give details, by all means do it, but you don't owe anyone information about your personal health choices.

GENDER REVEALS *

A lot of emphasis gets placed on genitals in our society, so people will wait with bated breath to hear the status of that fetal peen or vagine. Some people will even feel personally insulted if you refuse to reveal the sex. There are a lot of fun ways to do gender reveals, like pink or blue cake being cut into, or pink or blue vomit coming out of your mouth—whatever reflects your level of excitement about traditional gender roles!

* FYI, gender and sex are two different things. Maybe you could have a sex reveal party instead; that sounds way more exciting anyway.

F THE HATERS

Even though you're amazing and powerful, some people are going to hear your news and think, "Ew!" Maybe they don't like kids or had a bad childhood they don't want to be reminded of. Maybe they're jealous, or see your timeline for having kids as an attack on where they're at in *their* life. Your pregnancy can sometimes make people feel like they're losing you to your kid, or shatter the illusion that they were the center of your universe. Whatever their reasons for being turned off, these are not the people to lean on for emotional support, since they're processing their own emotions about what's happening to you. So just act pretty chill around them, as though having a smaller human in your care for the next eighteen years is NBD. Hopefully everyone reacts calmly to your news, but you'll get through this even if they don't.

· · · · · · · ·

At the end of the day, how you share your news and how people react to it doesn't really matter. So if you want to have fun with sharing your excitement, then have at it! This is all yours!

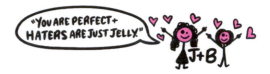

UGH, MATERNITY "FASHION"

As you expand, your clothing options narrow considerably, making it hard to feel fashionable, let alone comfortable. Here are some options that will hopefully wick away your sweat and your round ligament pain.

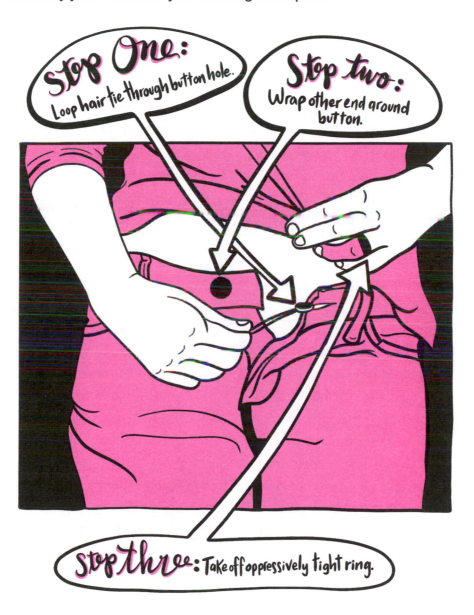

PANTS EXTENDERS

You'll learn quickly just how low the uterus sits in your pelvis, when that early belly is less bump and more FUPA.* Your upper vag will start busting out of your pants pretty early on, with the waistband feeling painfully restrictive. If your pants still fit otherwise, you may want to start rocking a pants extender. As glamorous as the name implies, this inelegant solution allows you to wear those pants just a little bit longer. These contraptions often leave your fly unzipped, so you'll need to pair with longer shirts if you don't want to look like you got chased out of a restroom mid-pee. If the thought of buying a pants extender is too depressing, try our hair tie trick.

MATERNITY PANTS

Eventually, even your loosest "bloat day" leggings will be too tight and you'll move on to a looser maternity pant (assuming you continue to wear pants at all). If your job requires you to look "presentable," it's probably worth investing in at least a couple of decent pairs. You have two basic choices here: under-the-bump or over-the-bump pants. Struggling to decide between two pretty terrible options? Ask yourself: Would you rather have a saggy butt or wear a full-body sock? The over-the-bump option will stay up better, keeping you warm in winter and exhaustingly, excruciatingly hot in summer. The under-the-bump option will have no "waist" to hold them on, so unless you have a true shelf of a booty, you'll have to constantly pull them back up onto your butt. Thankfully this not-a-sock version *doesn't* encase your pulsing body in tight Lycra with no breathability.

MATERNITY TOPS

Your choices will probably be limited to simple black and gray basics and a variety of grandmotherly florals. See what you can find online. Google "cool maternity clothes." Congrats—you're trying to be a "cool mom" in a world that doesn't believe that's a thing. Unfortunately, few retailers stock their maternity lines in physical stores for you to try on, assuming they even have a maternity line to begin with. Mumble curses toward the fashion industry and buy food instead.

FRILLY SHIT

Maternity clothes often come in a variety of pure whites, perky pinks, and soft grays. Designers decorate the expanding silhouettes with pleats and ruching that all add an extra layer of "maternal" to maternity. If you're

* Fat Upper Pelvic Area

into serving up "sweet little mommy" vibes, you're in luck! If you're not, buy six of the same "just okay" shirt in the same color.

YOUR PARTNER'S CLOTHES

If your partner is larger than you, you may want to borrow some of his or her clothes. If they're smaller than you, now is the time to start feeding them densely caloric foods.

COMFY SHOES

Your feet may spread and the arch may flatten under your increased weight. This means you may go up a shoe size, either temporarily or permanently. Your feet will be extra swollen in the last weeks of pregnancy, so find something comfy to wear, even if it means wearing slippers to work every day.

A WELL-FITTING BLACK OUTFIT

An all-black outfit is figure flattering, simple, streamlined, and severe. It says, "Don't talk to me about my body or I will eat you." It can also be easily accessorized with items from your prepregnancy life, like colorful cardigans, unbuttoned flannels, or chunky elephant jewelry, if that's your thing.

WHAT SIZE DO I EVEN BUY?

If you're not sure, buy bigger than your normal size. You'll thank us later. You may even need multiple sizes of maternity clothes over the course of your pregnancy. There is no shame in this. Buy clothing that makes you feel good when you can afford it and try to shrug it off when you can't. Repeat the mantra: "Every. Pregnancy. Ends!"

A MATERNITY BATHING SUIT YOU LOVE

Pregnancy and swimming are BF4E,* because as your belly grows, the relentless pull of gravity can really ruin your day. Floating in water is the ultimate relief, especially if you're heavily pregnant in summer. Don't be afraid to pick one of those hot two-piece numbers, either! It will be empowering to expose your gorgeous belly in public, and the sun feels amazing on itchy, tight belly skin. Bonus points if it's nursing-friendly so you can whip that titty out at the public pool in a few months.

* BeSt FrIeNdZ 4 EvA

GOOD BRAS THAT DON'T MAKE YOU WANT TO MURDER

Daaaamn, girl, them titties are slammin'! But seriously, your boobs are swelling up and will continue to do so. Your rib cage may also expand. Check in with yourself often to see if your bra is still feeling good, and replace it if it's pinchy or stabby. Put the old ones in a drawer for when you eventually start to deflate,* and get yourself to one of those crazy, old bra ladies who are always blowing everyone's mind. Try not to be offended when you walk in and show her your 36C boulder holder and she laughs in your face and hands you a 42A. They have a shtick, but they're very good at their job.

BELLY-SUPPORT BANDS/ CONTRAPTIONS

There are many levels of belly support, from the elastic band of your maternity jeans that hold up your tiny four-month bump, to vagina bras, to the industrial-grade Velcro behemoth that wraps up and around your boobs and makes loud scraping noises when you walk. The goal of all belly-support garments is to take some of the weight of your growing belly off your pelvic area in order to ease pain. Some women are completely fine without them, and some women graduate to more support several times as their pregnancy progresses. If you're feeling pain in your groin, don't wait; just go buy the ugly thing and put it on. Unfortunately, this is yet another area where the product that works for your friend may not be the best fit for you, so you may need to try more than one. Thankfully this pain will end soon after you give birth.

· · · · · · · · ·

If you can find them, you'll probably feel best in clothes that are similar to what you always wore; you don't *have* to look like a three-tier cake. No matter how uncomfortable this new body feels, try to find the emotional resources to not just *accept* yourself but really love yourself in all your glory. If there was ever a time for you to be okay with taking up space, that time is now. Your body is powerful. You are incredible. Fuck the patriarchy.

· · · · · · · · ·

* After pregnancy and/or breastfeeding, your breasts will shrink pretty dramatically. Enjoy your funbags while they last!

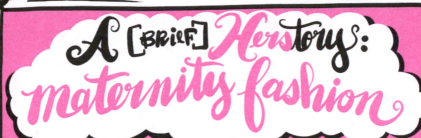

A [BRIEF] Herstory: maternity fashion

FOR MOST OF RECORDED HISTORY, PREGNANT WOMEN WERE PRETTY S.O.L. WHEN IT CAME TO FASHION. AS THE "ONE" DRESS YOU OWNED GOT TIGHTER, YOU COULD, UH... CUT IT? COVER THE GAP WITH YOUR APRON? HIDE IN THE ROOT CELLAR FOR A FEW MONTHS? HONESTLY, WOMEN WERE BASICALLY JUST PROPERTY BACK THEN, SO IT TOOK A LONG TIME TO FINALLY GET...

THE ADRIENNE DRESS: 1600s

The first maternity gown. The folds of the fabric were designed to expand with your growing belly. Like the rest of women's choices during this time it was heavy + oppressive, but it WAS bigger! Progress?

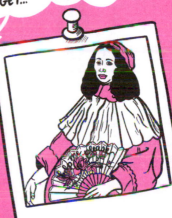

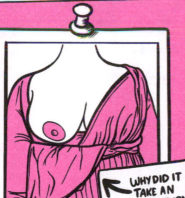

WHY DID IT TAKE AN ENTIRE CENTURY TO ADD THIS FLAP? #LISTEN2WOMEN

ADRIENNE "GETS SOME" – 1700s

~~Men~~ Babies could now more easily access women's breasts with a new removable "titty bib." Coincidentally, the first recorded incidence of public breastfeeding shaming also occurs around this time.

UNDER PRESSURE! 1800s

If you've ever stuffed your swollen sausage body into pregnancy Spanx, you will feel compassion for the plight of the Victorian preggo, who spent her long-AF days in a lace-up corset made of whale bones. Just like you, she pretended the corset "offered support" and "isn't too tight, just not feeling super hungry today."

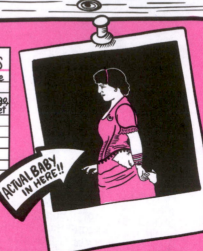

ACTUAL BABY IN HERE!!

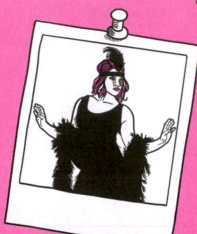

"NICE FLAPS!" — THE ROARING 20s!

After the Suffragette movement, women gained a bit more freedom. While the corsets and oppression continued pretty much unabated, showing leg was "in," now! During the 1920s women were given the opportunity to be newly objectified for their gusto + free will, perhaps b/c men were bored (PROHIBITION) and wanted to switch things up a little.

"LUCY IS ENCEINTE" → 1952

In this classic episode of "I Love Lucy," Lucille Ball makes history as the first woman to wear maternity clothes and be "openly pregnant" on TV. Until televised, pregnancy was an urban legend! After her debut, all expectant mothers were legally required to perm + dye their hair red.*

*THEY WERE LATER SHAMED FOR USING HAIR DYE WHILE PREGNANT.

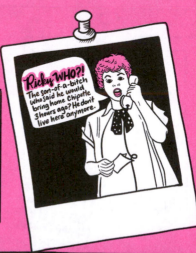

Ricky WHO?!
The son-of-a-bitch who said he would bring home Chipotle 3 hours ago? He don't live here anymore.

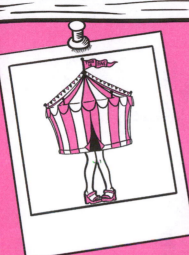

1950s – '90s → HIDE YO' SHAME!

Pinafores, tents + mumus for all! The fashion industry believed there was "no market" for interesting/comfortable maternity fashion, because women were obviously most interested in trying to hide how "fat" they were becoming.

"ACTUALLY NM, FLAUNT THAT BUMP!" – THE NiNeTiES!

As always, it was celebrities who reminded us what was truly important. As Hollywood actresses began to show us all how to be pregnant correctly, a baby bump became yet another thing you could dress "wrong."

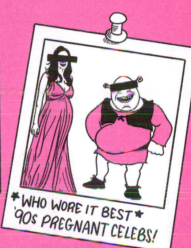

✻ WHO WORE IT BEST ✻
'90s PREGNANT CELEBS!

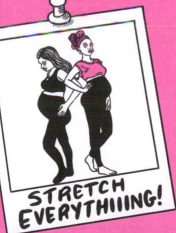

STRETCH EVERYTHIIING!

PRESENT DAY: ♡ ATHLEISURE ♡

CONGRATULATIONS!! Fate has selected you to live in the GOLDEN AGE of maternity fashion! Yoga pants and leggings both officially "count" as pants now, no matter what your creepy uncle mansplained last Thanksgiving. Athleisure is PREGNANT FREEDOM with an elastic waistband!

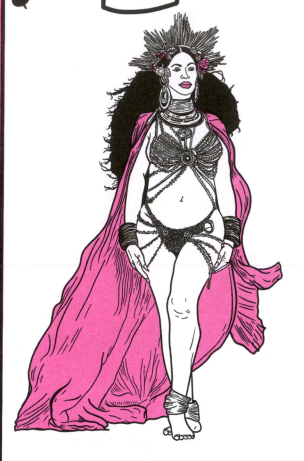

GOALS

*JK, THERE IS ONLY ONE BEYONCÉ.

WEIRD THIRD-TRIMESTER PREGNANCY SYMPTOMS

In addition to all the excitement and anticipation of your baby's looming arrival, in the third trimester, you're forced to contend with a slew of weirder and weirder pregnancy symptoms.

YOUR BOD'S CREAKIN'

As your joints loosen more and more, you may find yourself experiencing actual creaks as you move. Your body will shift and resettle like plates of the earth's crust. You may feel unsteady or in pain. You are like Mother Earth herself—powerful, angry, and ready to spew fire.

YOU HAVE "LIGHTNING CROTCH"?!

In the last days of pregnancy, particularly as your baby's head lowers into your pelvis, you may find yourself experiencing a new and specific crotch ache, especially after periods of standing, walking, or trying to retain some semblance of a normal human life. If you have pain in your pelvis, vulva, or rectum that is sharp and stabby, this is what health-care providers appropriately refer to as "lightning crotch." This may be caused by your baby's movements, a magnesium deficiency, actual varicose veins forming in your vagina, a posterior baby, or the stretching of round ligaments. You may find some relief via a chiropractor, acupuncture/acupressure, supportive clothing, magnesium supplements, exercises that help loosen the round ligament muscles, and screaming "Ow, fuck!" as often as possible.

YOUR THIGHS ARE CHAFIN'

If you're one of those special people who never experienced the infamous "chub rub," now may be your time! If you've already been there, it gets worse! Consider wearing shorts under dresses or lubing up with Vaseline or Body Glide.

YOU ALWAYS HAVE TO PEE

You now have to pee more often. This often starts early in pregnancy due to hormones, but once the baby's head is pressing on the bladder, you feel it all the time. And the occasional punch to the bladder can make you pee your pants. Fun! Pee before you leave the house, and then scout out every single possible pit stop along your commute. "Will I pee my pants today?" is a fun game you'll play. Consider wearing a panty liner, since you never know when you'll have a little accident, and also since you might be producing more discharge now that you're truly swole. Frequent urination can also be a sign of gestational diabetes, so it may be worth mentioning to your provider.

YOUR BOOBS OOZE

As they prepare for breastfeeding, your nipples might ooze strange yellowish liquid, which is early colostrum. You might find dried yellow bits on your nips or in your bra. You're getting ripe!

YOU HAVE STABBING RIB PAIN OUT OF THE BLUE

As your baby grows, they'll reach out into unexpected parts of you—a painful punch to your vagina or an unnervingly high kick to your chest. On the plus side, your growing frustration with pregnancy is one of the surest ways to overcome your fear of birth.

YOUR FARTS SMELL LIKE DEATH

As we've mentioned, your digestion is a hot mess right now. As your baby takes up more of the room meant for your intestines, food will stagnate inside you and your farts will reek like the bowels of hell. You have every right to continue farting in close proximity to offended family members as often as possible. You are a creator of life who giveth in many forms, and these mere mortals shall cower in your wake.

YOU SEEM EVEN *MORE* STONED

Most moms feel varying degrees of spaciness throughout pregnancy. But in the last month or so, the brain fog can really take over as you are transported to a mystical realm somewhere between earth and the other side. You're undergoing a lot, both physically and emotionally, as you process the insane life change on the horizon, so feel free to step out of your head for a while, even as you scramble to paint the baby's room or get ahead at work before your maternity leave. Whatever you're "supposed" to be doing can probably be done by someone who isn't conjuring life.

YOU'RE LITERALLY BIGFOOT

You're expanding, and your feet have to support that. Your feet and ankles may swell, especially if you've been walking or standing. This can be painful. So put your feet up when you can. Cash in some pregnancy pity points and make your partner rub your feet. You deserve it, like every other pleasure, but especially because a zero-cost, zero-calorie foot rub is guilt-free. Make your partner read this chapter, and then make them rub your feet.

I Slept Like a Baby

(Was Inside Me)

Despite pregnancy exhaustion, you may find sleep harder to achieve than ever. Babies often sleep to the comforting jostle of your movements throughout the day, which means the stillness of night is their time to play. And by play, we mean hurt you from the inside. Plus, now that your stomach is an extra appendage, it's difficult to find a comfortable position. Sleeping on your belly is dangerous, and sleeping on your back is somehow also dangerous.

Your hips will ache, and unless you prop yourself up on a bunch of pillows, your stomach acid may creep into your throat, giving you a raging heartburn. Oh, also, from time to time you will wake up with a hunger like you've never felt before. Here are some . . .

Fun Ways Not to Sleep

* Drink or eat within a few hours of bedtime (because you are a hungry pregnant lady) and get heartburn as soon as you lie down.

* Don't drink or eat before bed in order to avoid heartburn and instead lie awake starving.

* Toss and turn trying to find a position that feels good.

* Find one fave position that then becomes excruciating as your body compresses onto the one joint supporting you.

* Lay awake thinking about the overwhelming weight of being responsible for another human.

* Endure the energetic activities of a seven-pound person who is eager to be outside of you.

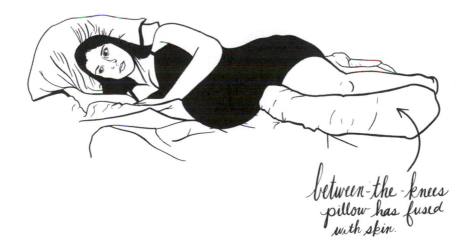

between-the-knees pillow has fused with skin.

YOU'RE FULL OF OTHER MYSTERIOUS PAINS

Something in your bones isn't right. You don't know what. Nothing seems to fix it. Health-care professionals will shrug and describe it as typical pregnancy pain, the possible stretching of ligaments. If men were pregnant, they would have a better answer. If you've exhausted your medical options, your best bet is to calculate the number of weeks you have left and try to feel optimistic about that number. Years from now you'll realize your rib was actually popping out of place slightly due to all the relaxin hormone. Oh well.

YOU MAY CRY FLOODS AND FLOODS OF TEARS

As your body continues to ripen and your hormones overflow you, you're probably going to feel emotional. And regardless of who is there to support you, at some point you're going to resent the fact that all of this is resting on your shoulders (and other joints). If you find yourself crying in surges, that's probably pretty normal. Do seek professional help if you're feeling overwhelmed. And if you don't have the capacity to hunt down resources, find someone close to you who will. Seriously. But if you just need a little cry followed by a Popsicle, that's cool too.

YOU FEEL SOMETHING LIKE A HOT FLASH

The end of pregnancy (particularly in warmer months) can make you feel very hot. We know we've said it a lot, but again—the hormones, the blood, the extra weight you're carrying around—everything is making your body run on overdrive. You may experience waves of heat that overwhelm you. If you feel a tensing of your back and abdominal muscles, these may be Braxton-Hicks contractions. If you're not super close to your due date, it's best to try to alleviate and prevent contractions by staying hydrated and avoiding aggressive physical activities. Let your health-care provider know if this is happening.

. . . .

Congrats—you're nearing the finish line of pregnancy! Most of this weird body stuff is less serious than it seems, and the memory will fade once you experience a baby coming out of your body. But for now, we feel your pain!

Pregnancy Sex

Your sexual interest during pregnancy is entirely unpredictable and may be impacted by various factors, including hormones, energy levels, stage of pregnancy, and how much you hate your partner on a given day. Some women who loved sex before pregnancy hate it while pregnant, and some women find themselves loving it like never before. That said, pregnancy sex is not without its challenges. Here are some aspects to consider.

CLITORAL PLEASURE IS YOUR FRIEND

Some find penetrative sex painful during pregnancy. Your pelvic area is more engorged, and the uterus is sitting lower, allowing less room for a penis, hand, or toy. So this may be a good time to lean into oral sex and smaller handheld toys that stimulate the clitoris. Both options require less maneuvering of your big pregnant body, while vibrating toys allow your partner to also be lazy if they're tired of putting in all the "elbow" grease. And if pregnancy is really amping up your sex drive, toys are great for solo play when your partner doesn't have the energy to meet your aggressive needs.

One weird fact about cunnilingus during pregnancy is that it is dangerous for your partner to blow air into your vagina, because it could force air into the bloodstream (though why they would attempt this, we have no idea). So don't let him or her literally blow you.

ORGASMS ARE DIFFERENT

Some women find that they are able to have multiple orgasms for the first time during pregnancy. So if you're down, why not give it a go? In the later stages of pregnancy, you may find your orgasms are different in a bad way. They might be kind of painful, or not as satisfying, and you may have cramping afterward. This does not mean anything is physically wrong with you or the baby. It just means that you have grown too powerful sexually, like some kind of bloated sex-Hulk.

Don't let anyone tell you that you should be any more or less sexual than you are feeling in any given moment. This is your body, your rules, and whatever your rules, you rule.

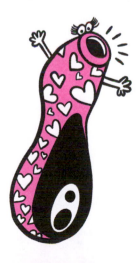

Weird Symptoms that Mean You Should Call Your Doctor/Midwife

* Liquid is coming out of your vagina (that isn't pee)

* Blood is coming out of your vagina

* Contractions (belly/back tightness or pain) every five minutes or less

* Constant severe pain

* Sudden swelling (fingers, feet, or face)

* Cloudy or stinky pee

* You can't remember the last time your baby moved inside you

* Blurry or impaired eyesight

* Persistent head pain

* Pain or redness in your leg

* Anything else that seems weird to you. There is never a wrong time to call your provider, even if he or she is the type who always brushes off your concerns and refers to you as a "healthy young woman."

Swelling, changes in vision, and some of the other symptoms listed could be signs of preeclampsia, a condition characterized by high blood pressure, water retention, and protein in the urine. Untreated, it can lead to seizures. While preeclampsia can be treated and carefully monitored, the only cure is delivering your baby, so if you're diagnosed, your provider may want to induce you early.

BABY SHOWERS!

Your baby shower / mother blessing is a very special event celebrating the last time in your life you will ever be the center of attention, unless you get a terminal illness. It's your time to shine before you slink gracefully into the shadow of your adorable baby for the foreseeable future.

The lesser-known mother blessing is loosely based on but trying very hard to be respectful of a Navajo rite of passage that celebrates a woman's transition into motherhood. If you haven't heard of it before, you're probably not a hippie! Motherhood is a great time to dip your toe into the granola pool—caftans and elastic-waist pants are the friend of hippie and pregnant woman alike, and essential oil diffusers are hip *and* useful.

A mother blessing is traditionally attended by the closest women in your life. It's a time to offer wisdom, give love and support, and welcome a woman into the generous folds of motherhood. Modern American culture focuses so much on the baby and baby products, but the transition into motherhood is one of the most profound experiences of life, which some would say deserves

BABY SHOWER	MOTHER BLESSING
CELEBRATES YOUR BABY!	**CELEBRATES YOU!**
Most guests bring presents for the baby/sometimes you.	Guests are sometimes asked to bring a small bead to contribute to a birthing necklace that will be made for your labor, so that you can be reminded of all the women supporting you and also look a little bananas as you labor.
People you love make you wear a trash "crown" on your head after opening your presents.	People you love offer you wisdom and also wash your feet in a fancy bowl with nice soap, if you want.
Might make you question our materialistic culture while also enjoying all the free stuff.	Might make you question "Is this cultural appropriation?" while also enjoying the connection to your community.

to be celebrated and honored just as much as cute onesies.

Some women choose to have only one of these events, and many have both or a combination of the two.

If you *do* choose to have a mother blessing and are not native, be respectful of traditions. Women can honor and lift up the ideas of other cultures (especially those who do a much better job at caring for their women) without appropriating those cultures for our own gain. Consider asking your guests to donate to a nonprofit in America that serves the native community and pay it forward.

YOUR SHOWER REGISTRY

Registering for presents enables you to completely control your baby's aesthetic, while not having to talk to anyone with your mouth. Tons of stores have their own registries, but you can also use a web service that will allow you to register for things at any store, which is much less complicated, unless you plan to buy literally everything at Target, which is a legit plan, in all honesty.

WHO TO INVITE

It's your party, and you'll mix lots of incompatible personalities from different parts of your life if you want to. Like a wedding, a baby shower is a time when all people from all corners of your life come together to make awkward conversation and eat crudité. Invite anyone and everyone you want, especially the rich relatives who want to buy your baby expensive swaddles.

WHAT TO WEAR

Since baby showers tend to happen toward the end of a pregnancy, comfort and easy access for peeing are key. Wear something that makes you feel cute but is still comfy AF.

WHAT TO DO

At some point, whoever is planning your shower will ask, "Do you want to play games?" What they are really asking is: "Do you want to lick melted candy bars out of a hot diaper and try to guess which kind of candy bar it is?" Well, do you? There are no wrong answers. Also, opening gifts is not required.

Opening gifts during a party is not fun for *anyone* involved, and you do not have to do it just because your mom wants you to open the stroller system she got you in front of a large crowd. Opening presents for an audience makes most gift recipients feel weird and greedy for no reason, makes your friends and family bored AF, makes the people who didn't bring a gift embarrassed, and forces your poor best friend/mom/aunt to spend half the party taking very detailed notes with a golf pencil on a scrap of wrapping paper so you can theoretically write personal and thoughtful thank-you notes later. Speaking of which . . .

THANK-YOU NOTES

Girl, all power to you if you're the kind of person who enjoys doing this (and also, welcome to Earth, supreme being!). If you're not though, just send a group text about how swollen and painful your pregnant hands are, and include a photo. Use an internet stock photo, if necessary, and humble-brag about saving trees and going "paperless." Motherhood has really made you more in touch with the earth, huh? You're so grounded.

BABY SHOWER = TIME TO GET HELP!

Your baby shower is not just about gifts and cake and mortifying games, it's also about turning your friends and family into temporary staff members. Leave a laptop open during the party so people can sign up to deliver you a meal, come sit with the baby while you shower, take the baby on a walk so you can nap, or smother you with a pillow when you can't take the colic for another fucking second, you just cannot.

Hot tip: Make your baby shower coed because you're a modern damn woman, and also because you can send the men to the baby room and make them put furniture together while you complain about them. When women stop doing so much emotional labor, men can stop being given manual labor tasks by default. Deal?

WHAT YOU ACTUALLY NEED TO OWN

Baby Clothes

You'll need many clothes in various sizes, factoring for lots of soiled clothing changes and speedy growth. Used clothing is *more* than acceptable. Things that are easy to get on and off are ideal.

Diapers

You'll need an infinite amount. Be ready to outgrow the newborn size within the first pack of diapers.

Something for Your Baby to Sleep In / Be Put Down In

A bassinet is fine. Babies tend to prefer bouncy chairs and things where they can be both upright and snuggled tightly into, but experts recommend they don't sleep in these things unattended overnight, so you'll also need a bassinet or crib. Unfortunately they will outgrow the bassinet very quickly.

Baby Monitor

You don't *need* one. But if it saves you one trip to get up and see what that weird gurgle noise is, it's probably worth it.

Swaddles

The fancy ones are easier to use than the plain old receiving blankets, but if you're on a budget, you can figure those out. Your baby might hate them all, but most babies like being wrapped up tight for the first month or so, as it reminds them of being inside you. It'll be very worth it to get them to stay asleep without being on top of you.

Sleep Sacks

Sleep sacks keep babies warm, like a blanket, but their arms are free, and unlike a blanket, they can't pull it up onto their face and suffocate. If you live somewhere cold, it's a pretty good idea to have one.

Burp Cloths

You'll need way more burp cloths than you think, since babies spit up roughly every three minutes. Towels are adequate, but a burp cloth will really absorb so that the mess doesn't drip onto your shirt. If you're breastfeeding, you'll also need some to shove down one side of your bra while your baby's nursing on the other side, since her feeding will trigger your letdown and cause the other boob to leak.

CONTROVERSIAL REGISTRY ITEMS

Baby-product opinions are like grandparents: everyone has them, and they are usually very gender-binary. Here are a few products that might elicit a response should you register for them, but also might greatly help you in your parenting journey.

Crib Bumpers

Some people believe these glorified fabric strips are the only way to keep your precious child from getting their legs stuck between the slats of the crib or smashing their poor little head, while others believe they will cause instant suffocation death. "But are the mesh ones okay????" you will scream into the void at 3:00 a.m., swollen with child and indecision. You will receive no answer.

Walkers

They might be *called* walkers, but what if your child never walks on their own because you put them in this lazy-making device that makes it too easy for them, and then they must use a walker for their whole entire life? Do you even know where to get a giant walker like that? Will it fit through doorways?

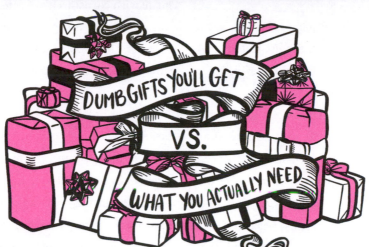

DUMB GIFTS YOU'LL GET VS. WHAT YOU ACTUALLY NEED

YOU'LL GET:

WHY?

WIPES WARMER

6 OF THESE THINGS?

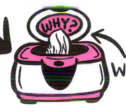

A FANCY SILVER RATTLE FOR BABY'S FIRST BLUDGEONING

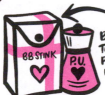

BB STINK

P.U.

BABY COLOGNE TO COVER UP THAT PUTRID NEWBORN BABY SMELL?

YOU NEED:

UNIVERSAL MATERNITY LEAVE POLICIES

BETTER POSTPARTUM HEALTH-CARE PRACTICES

RECOGNITION OF THE LABOR CAPITAL OF STAY-AT-HOME MOMS

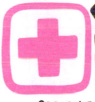
= PAY

$ $ AFFORDABLE CHILD CARE $

WE HOPE YOU KEPT THOSE GIFT RECEIPTS! ♥

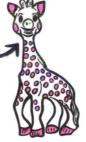
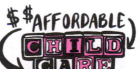

Disposable Diapers

The cloth diaper movement is a great way to be environmentally conscious, but it's not realistic for everyone. Cloth diapering is initially more expensive (you need to build your "stash" and have some equipment and cleaning supplies), and much more time-consuming. Additionally, many daycare centers will not change cloth diapers. Despite these roadblocks, women are still shamed for using disposable diapers, because you're not just responsible for mothering your child but also for saving the planet!

Teething Medicine

Teething is a natural (torturous) process, so giving your baby medicine is often frowned upon. Menstruation is also a natural process, and it hurts like a bitch and drugs are good. Teething medicine given according to the directions on the package will allow your baby to sleep, and that is a very good thing. Do your own research and talk to your pediatrician and decide what you're comfortable with, and try to ignore fearmongering from "concerned" relatives and other parents.

Baby Powder

Our moms pretty much breaded us in talcum powder, but studies now show a correlation to ovarian cancer. Thanks, Mom! Powders made with cornstarch are safer, *for now, anyway*. Honestly, it's pretty important to remember that you're going to fuck this up somehow no matter how hard you try.

Anything Magnetic

Magnets will kill your baby!!! They will swallow two magnets and the magnets will stick together in some crucial part of their internal organ system and it will kill them. It's best to have a strict magnet policy in your home and to inform visitors in writing before they enter. Magnetic onesies are okay though, because they are *so easy* to change in the middle of the night. Also those fridge magnets of letters and numbers are so cute and useful while you're cooking. You know what, just watch your baby and make sure they don't eat the magnets. It's probably fine.

Blue Clothing for Girls

Very quickly after your child is born, you will notice that it seems very important that strangers are able to correctly identify the gender of your child. They will say things like "Awwwww, what a beautiful little . . . girl?" They will expect you to cooperate and identify your child as a woman so that they may begin oppressing her appropriately. If you do decide to dress your daughter in blue, maybe pierce her ears for the sake of confused strangers? She will cry now, but she will thank you later when she's a cruising toddler in big gold summer hoops.

Pink Clothing for Boys

HOW DARE YOU! Don't you know how uncomfortable that's going to make your crazy old relatives? It's okay, they'll all be dead soon. *Wink.*

Stuff for You

Nah, girl, that's not controversial. You deserve those microwavable soothing tit pillows. Times are hard. Register for things that will make your life easier and make your body feel better. You deserve it, queen.

People at your baby shower often feel that this is their chance to weigh in on your parenting choices, because their opinions *need to be heard*! Remember, this is your baby and your celebration, and if you have any truly toxic friends or relatives, just "forget" to invite them, saying, "Sorry, we were so busy getting ready for the baby, we just threw together a really teensy tiny party of a few friends at the last minute."

Some Things You Are Now Legally Required to Make by Hand

Oh, did you think that making a baby with your body was more than enough to call yourself a mother? Wrong. Mothers are meant to be goddesses of creation, crafting everything their family could ever dream of owning. Choke down that acid reflux and get to work on your Pinterest board full of handmade, eco-friendly stuffies, tiny banners, and a baby keepsake book to remain empty and haunt you for the rest of your life. IT'S THE LAW.

YOUR FIRST KNITTING PROJECT EVER: A SQUARISH HAT (?)

There's a reason why old women are so good at knitting: they are old. If you make a pregnant decision to take up the art of weaving with small sticks, you will probably not be very good at first. Keep up your third attempt at a hat though. You'll be proud of it when you put it on your kid, whose head shape is going to be very strange at first, anyway.

A FREEZER FULL OF HOME-COOKED RECIPES EVEN THOUGH YOU PRETTY MUCH NEVER COOK ANYMORE AND ORDER CHEESECAKE EVERY NIGHT FROM THAT SHITTY PLACE ON GRUBHUB

Every baby-prep list includes this tip—"Stock your freezer with home-cooked meals that can be easily portioned out." Although no human woman fully enjoys eating freezer food, having food readily available in the first few months of your child's life is a pretty good idea. Some people even purchase a chest freezer, which is also helpful for storing breast milk if you plan to pump and never stop pumping. Some people also buy chest freezers because they hunt deer, just something to consider as you develop your momdentity. Above all, remember this—if you end up ordering takeout later, rather than eating some freezer-burned bullshit lasagna, no one is going to blame you.

AN INSPIRATIONAL BANNER TO HANG ABOVE YOUR ILLITERATE INFANT'S CRIB

Think of it this way: How do you *know* your baby can't read? What if he can, and there's no pennant above his bed assuring him that you *Love Him to the Moon and Back*? It's ageist to assume that your child can't read just because he has never told you he can. Make the pennant—it's important.

TINY STICKERS TO PUT ON THE BABY'S SQUIRMING BODY FOR INSTAGRAM MONTHLIES

The first seven to eight months of a baby's life are monotonous. There's a lot of shushing and patting and droopy heads and crying and spaced-out-gurgle-smiling, which can take a toll on overall mental sharpness. Babies change slowly; your baby's four- and five-month photos will be mostly indistinguishable but for the sticker on her duck pajamas, so it's

best to clearly label your work for future reference. Go ahead and print all twelve stickers, but we give you three months of keeping up this exhausting charade. Once you start posting them a few days late, it's a slippery slope.

PARTNER CHORE CHART

Just a few years ago, you cleaned only when people besides your best friend were coming over, but now you are a hormonal beast who hates dirt, perpetually wiping down kitchen counters. If you want to continue loving your partner after birth, you will need to delegate. There are lots of apps that do this, but you're pregnant, so you will need to do arts and crafts. Hang your chore chart somewhere where you'll see it often, and use washi tape[*] because #instagramworthy.

PLACENTA ART

You grew it for nine months; it'd be a shame to just throw it away! The final opus of your pregnancy is birth, and what you do with your placenta is your artist's statement. Some women choose to have it dried and encapsulated into pills that they ingest postpartum; this is called performance art. Others press the still-pulsing space organ into paper to create a print and then roll it up and put it in a closet for many years. Whatever you choose, remember that your body created your placenta to feed and protect your child while it grew inside of you, and it is *way* bigger than you imagined it being.

* Colorful, more expensive tape

WHEN YOU WANT TO SCREAM

Pregnancy causes a *lot* of stress and anxiety. Not only is your life about to become completely different, but your body is going through a horror movie transformation. You'll lie awake wondering if you're ready to have a child and whether you've already somehow ruined it. You'll wonder how this baby will impact the career that is helping you afford to have a baby in the first place. You'll conduct nonstop assessments of your partner's parenting ability. You'll think "What am I doing?" as you recount your family health history. And everyone will be staring at your body *all of the time!*

If you're feeling unusually stressed, talk to your provider and/or therapist. If it's run-of-the-mill, "I keep getting bigger while my world is shrinking around me" anxiety, try to breathe. Everything is going to work out, and you're going to be a great mom.

Things to Think About If You're Trying to Think of Something to Worry About

- "Do people think I'm going to be a good mom even though I was really late to a party once?"

- "Will my baby have short legs like me?"

- "Should I brainstorm more baby names since the initials I've currently settled on spell TUD and that looks kind of dumb?"

- "How many towels should I keep in the car just in case I give birth in there? Should I just do paper towels?"

- "Am I eating enough almonds?"

RELATIONSHIP STRESS

There are a lot of ways your partner can stress you out during pregnancy. One way is if you don't feel like they're helping you prepare. Conversely, your pregnancy can also flip a switch in your partner's brain that causes them to think deeply about their role as provider, causing them to stress you out about things you don't want to think about right now, like money, logistics, and whether they'll still be allowed to take beer-making classes. Now's a good time to start setting boundaries and expectations with your partner. So feel free to say things like . . .

- "I'm tired and pregnant and don't want to hear about that right now."

- "If I can make you a child, you can figure out how to cook meatballs."

- "I *will* spend eight hundred dollars on a doula unless you can tell me what a rebozo is."

WHAT TO DO WHEN YOU NEED A GOOD CRY

Over the course of your pregnancy, there will be moments when your emotions run *high AF* and moments when you feel plugged up and desperate for the sweet release of some old-fashioned "face rain." When the tears aren't flowing, here are some emotional roller coasters to help you get blubbering, *fast*.

Visit the SPCA

Roam through the stalls and let the sweet little puppies and kittens nuzzle your hand through the bars. Each one of these animals was once a baby, and now they are alone and afraid. **IMPORTANT: DO *NOT* GET A PET WHILE YOU ARE PREGNANT.**

Look at Baby Pictures of You with Your Mom

Hoo boy. Good relationship with your mom? You're gonna sob. Bad relationship? Girrrrrl, you're gonna sob hard. Seeing your mom as a tender young mother will make you relate to her in a way you haven't before and will make you remember your mortality, and hers. Tear City, USA, population: you! And her, if you text her one.

Watch the Following Videos

- Baby Animals Being Born

  The stoic calm of a mama giraffe as she births her calf takes on a whole new level of meaning when you're swollen with your own little calf. Didn't do the trick? Do a trust fall into the rabbit hole of animal videos and you're sure to find a winner. That sneezing panda one? Come on. Let yourself go.

- High-Budget Birthing Flicks

  The nitty-gritty ones are also great to watch, but if you're trying to rub out a quick sob, you want Tessa's Home Birth Journey *or* The Gentle Earthside Coming of Solar Rayplex *or one of the countless professionally shot and edited "birth films."*

- *Lemonade*

  So many reasons to cry here! Can you relate to Beyoncé as a woman scorned?

The fact that her literal masterpiece of a full visual album was ignored by critics because she's a black woman? Or the fact that in the end, she still loves Jay-Z and forgives him? Or just feeling emotional knowing that she too has been pregnant? Stop, it's too much.

Read Today's Newspaper

Just read anything at all about our heartbreakingly terrible and beautiful world.

· · · · · · · ·

Forget what the patriarchy told you—being "emotional" isn't a bad thing. In fact, it's a good thing. It's called "emotional release" for a reason. So let 'er rip!

GETTING YOUR BODY READY FOR BIRTH

As your due date approaches, there are some extra things you can do in order to get your body into tip-top shape for shooting out a person.

RED RASPBERRY LEAF TEA

In the third trimester, red raspberry leaf tea is recommended to improve uterine muscle tone and prepare the body for labor. This can help give your body stronger, more efficient contractions, which in turn may reduce the need for medical intervention. It is also said to boost milk production in breastfeeding moms. Unfortunately, it tastes pretty meh.

PROBIOTICS

Probiotics may help prevent you testing positive for a Group B strep infection. Group B streptococcus is a bacteria found in the vagina or rectum of 25 percent of healthy adult women. It's normally not a problem; however, you risk passing the bacteria to your baby during birth, which could cause complications. Therefore women who test positive for strep B will be given antibiotics during birth. This isn't a big deal, except that antibi-

otics have minor side effects you might want to avoid, especially in addition to other drugs you might be given during labor. So take probiotic pills or eat foods like kefir that are rich in probiotic strains. This will also help with pregnancy constipation, which can hit hardest in late pregnancy.

VAGINA STRETCHING

You may want to prep your vagina for delivery in order to prevent or minimize vaginal tears. The EPI-NO is a balloon device you insert in your vagina and inflate in order to stretch it over time. It can be painful and annoying and is definitely not for everyone, but it does train your vagina to stretch, give you a sense of what you're in for, and an excuse to practice breathing exercises. The EPI-NO is difficult to obtain in the United States since it is not FDA approved, but it can often be procured internationally via a midwife. An alternative method of preventing tears is perineal massage, which is where you or your partner massage your perineum with oil. Why not, right?! Oh, you're tired? Hmm.

MONITORING YOUR BABY'S POSITION

If you're not already planning a C-section, your doctor or midwife will often check your baby's position to see how it might affect

What the Heck Is a Contraction, Really?

A contraction is the tightening and then releasing of the uterus muscle, which squeezes the uterus in a wavelike motion from top to bottom. This may feel like a tightening or hardening of your stomach, very intense menstrual-like cramps or back pain, sometimes accompanied by pressure on the pelvis.*

The weaker, irregular contractions you might feel in the weeks prior to going into labor are called **Braxton-Hicks** contractions. You will know these contractions are not "true" labor because there will be no discernible pattern to their frequency and they will not get stronger or closer together over time. Real labor contractions will not stop if you change position or relax, but Braxton-Hicks contractions can often be stopped by resting, getting up and moving, or drinking lots of water. Labor contractions will open your cervix while shrinking the size of your uterus smaller and smaller, forcing your baby out of you.

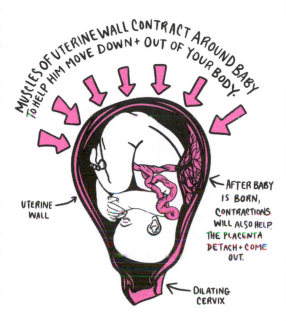

MUSCLES OF UTERINE WALL CONTRACT AROUND BABY TO HELP HIM MOVE DOWN + OUT OF YOUR BODY.

UTERINE WALL

AFTER BABY IS BORN, CONTRACTIONS WILL ALSO HELP THE PLACENTA DETACH + COME OUT.

DILATING CERVIX

* * * * * * * *

* For more on what contractions feel like and how to time them, see "The Start, Stop, Wait," page 126.

WHAT IS CERVICAL RIPENING?

Cervical ripening or cervical effacement is when your cervix softens, shortens, and thins. This may begin in the hours or days before your labor has begun. This process readies your cervix to dilate (open) during labor.

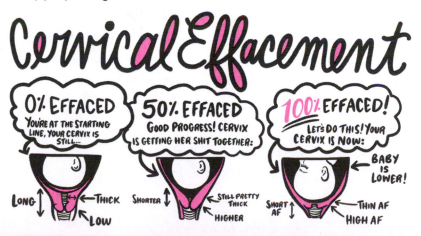

Cervical Effacement

0% EFFACED
YOU'RE AT THE STARTING LINE, YOUR CERVIX IS STILL...
LONG
THICK
LOW

50% EFFACED
GOOD PROGRESS! CERVIX IS GETTING HER SHIT TOGETHER:
SHORTER
STILL PRETTY THICK
HIGHER

100% EFFACED!
LET'S DO THIS! YOUR CERVIX IS NOW:
BABY IS LOWER!
SHORT AF
THIN AF
HIGH AF

your birth later. If your baby is breech (head near your chest, feet near your vagina), you may not be able to deliver vaginally. And if your baby is facing forward, it may result in back labor.* Sometimes the baby's position will correct on its own over the last few weeks of pregnancy, especially if you're doing preventative measures like the ones we'll mention next. Ask your doula or midwife to teach you how to feel your baby's position. You can tell the baby's head and butt apart by how hard they are. You can also grab either with your hand and wiggle—you'll know it's the butt if the whole baby moves with it, whereas the head will wiggle independently from the body. (Don't worry—this is less harmful than it seems!)

YOGA, MOVEMENT, AND POSTURE

Since many of us spend a lot of time sitting, our posture and hip alignment can be a bit off, making it harder to squeeze out a baby. Light exercises like walking or yoga can help alignment. Cat-cow pose,† also known as pelvic tilts (or any activity where you are on your hands and knees), can help spin the baby in the right direction. You can also sit on a yoga

ball or lean forward in your chair during the day so that your knees and belly are lower than your hips. Here are some helpful exercises for positioning the baby. Talk to your doctor or midwife before attempting, especially if you have health conditions.

Forward-Leaning Inversion

Kneel on the edge of a couch or low bed, carefully lowering your hands to the floor. Rest your weight on your elbows and let your head hang loosely, keeping your back flat. Sway your hips, if it feels good. Stay here for thirty seconds, taking three slow deep breaths, and then push yourself back up onto your knees.

Windmill

Stand with your feet wider than hip-width apart. On an inhale, reach up through the crown of your head to make yourself as tall as possible. On your exhale, lean forward, placing your hands on the ground or on a support like yoga blocks if that feels more comfortable. On your next inhale, lift one arm up over your head as you look up at it. Exhale and bring the arm back down and switch arms.

* * * * * * * * *
* For more on back labor, see "The Weirdness of Labor," page 130.
† See "A 'Healthy' Pregnancy," page 18, for a how-to.

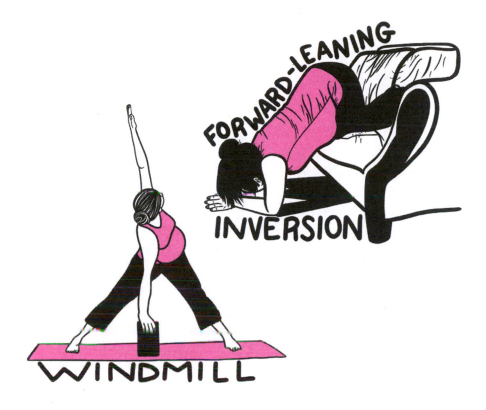

WINDMILL

FORWARD-LEANING INVERSION

CHIROPRACTOR

Another way to improve alignment is by visiting a chiropractor. If you're not sure your hip joints are moving properly, it may be worth a visit to find out. Again, this is particularly worthwhile if you are planning to labor without medication and hope to avoid a C-section.

REST

Take it easy! Put up those achy feet! This is your last chance to nap when you wanna nap and watch TV for an entire day. It's like your life has been one long summer vacation that's about to end any moment, so milk every second.

· · · · · · · ·

You'll never really know if you needed any of this shit, but you may find yourself wishing you'd tried it later. Do what feels right, without overloading yourself mentally, physically, or financially. Good luck!

PREGNANCY AND BIRTH TERMS THAT IT'S TIME TO RETIRE

In pregnancy we're introduced to a myriad of confusing terms, many of which just don't seem right. Let's pin the failure of this squarely on the men, who no doubt labeled our bodies this way, and retire the following terms.

"BREAST IS BEST"

A phrase once meant to empower women who chose to breastfeed, it's now become associated with the shaming of women who don't. Some are replacing it with the term "fed is best," which recognizes that many women deal with factors that prevent them from breastfeeding or wanting to attempt it. While we don't discount the health benefits of breastfeeding, it's time for this term to go. The language describing our choices should not divide us into winners and losers.

"CERVIX"

Ask anyone who hasn't been pregnant and they may not even know what a cervix is.

Sure, the ignorance surrounding female anatomy is the failure of our country's education system, which spends an inordinate amount of time focused on male sperm, but maybe if we rebranded this "magical sphincter" it would get a little more attention. Maybe we should call it "the baby portal." Because "cervix" sounds like something you'd use to get rid of your dog's mite infestation.

"CERVICAL RIPENING"

Nope.

"DUE DATE"

Unless you schedule a C-section, there's no way of knowing exactly when you'll deliver. First-time moms, on average, deliver about a week later than their due date. Some women prefer the term "guess date"; it takes the pressure off in those excruciating final days of pregnancy, when some would refer to you as "overdue."[*] Girl, you're not a library book.

"FUNDAL HEIGHT"

A term for how high the top of your uterus (fundus) is in your body, used to make you nervous that your belly is growing too quickly or too slowly. Doesn't sound very *fun, dus it*?[†]

[*] Or to put it more kindly, "fashionably late."

[†] Sorry.

"GERIATRIC PREGNANCY" OR "ADVANCED MATERNAL AGE"

"Geriatric pregnancy" is a term used by doctors to describe a woman who becomes pregnant over the age of thirty-five. This is 100 percent a term invented by a man. A woman of normal childbearing age should not be labeled elderly. At some point some people realized this and started using the term "advanced maternal age," as if that's really any better. If we must characterize expectant moms over thirty-five, how about "she can still get it" pregnancies, or "major MILF over here."

"MECONIUM"

Meconium sounds like a newly discovered radioactive element or a superhero's archnemesis. But actually it's just your baby's first poop. Let's call it "new poop" or maybe just "the black poop." Imagine how much more sense it would make if your doctor said, "Your baby did a sticky poop into the water he's been living in, so we're gonna suck some goop out of his mouth because inhaling poop could fuck up his breathing" instead of the more enigmatic "there's meconium in your amniotic fluid, so we're going to use suction."

"MUCUS PLUG"

The name is as gross as this thing is to look at, but does it have to be? It might be nice if one of the first signs of labor wasn't described like something a plumber fished out of your drain.

" 'LOSING' YOUR MUCUS PLUG" OR "THE BLOODY SHOW"

No one loses their mucus plug; we flush it down the toilet. We know exactly where it went and chose to dispose of it, because we are not hoarders. And "bloody show" sounds like the kind of show we never, ever want to see.

"NATURAL BIRTH"

There is no type of birth that is more "natural" than another. Whether a woman delivers vaginally or via C-section, she made a human being with her body, and that baby is as earthly as the rest of us, not some "unnatural" creation. The term "natural birth" contributes to stigma around necessary medical care that many women undergo to save the lives of themselves and/or their babies. So let's stop saying we had a "natural birth" as if other women didn't. The preferred term is "unmedicated birth."

"OBSTETRICS"

This isn't a crossword puzzle—it's a woman's body. How 'bout "womb studies" or something witchy like "watching life."

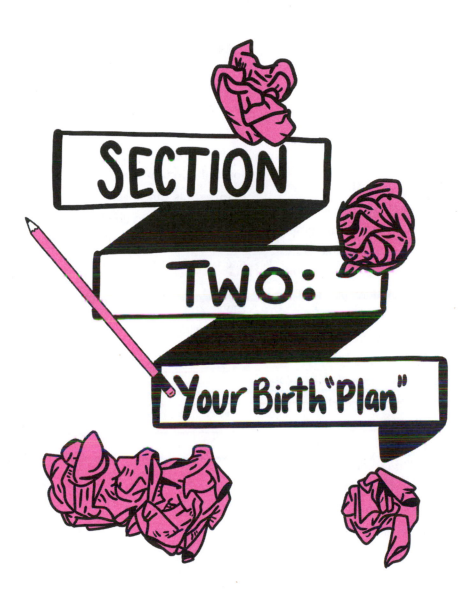

SECTION TWO:

"Your Birth "Plan""

HOW TO PLAN THE PERFECT BIRTH FOR YOUR BABY TO RUIN

Here's the thing about birth plans: babies don't give a fuuuuuck about birth plans. Don't get us wrong: you should have one. You should be well prepared for the birth you want, but a lot of times plans change. Sometimes you get the dreamy orgasmic water birth you dreamed of having, or the perfectly timed epidural you had nightmares about not happening, and other times you end up shooting out a baby into your yoga pants in a cab on the way to the hospital. Any "plan" you have for your child's birth will be thrown out the window once your labor starts to unfold in real time. Still, it's good to research your options and likely scenarios so that you have some sense of how you want it to go down. It'll be harder to make these decisions when your knees are pressed to your chest and an unseen force is seizing at the core of your being. Your partner may also want to think about their own role and whether they'd like to cut the

cord, so that they don't freeze up and babble "Wuwuwuh?" like a cartoon duck when a nurse presents them with what looks like a bloody entrail.

Even if literally nothing goes as planned, having an ideal scenario helps your support team figure out what to prioritize in addition to any obvious medical needs of you and your child. Your perfect scenario may end up thwarted as unexpected factors present themselves and the blinding reality of contractions becomes tangible. Childbirth is one of the most humbling experiences life can throw at you (aside from accidentally showing up to the advanced workout class) and a fitting entrée to your unruly new life. Try to go with the flow, because the flow may be very much like a tsunami.

SHUTTING DOWN YOUR BIRTH-PLAN HATERS

As we've mentioned throughout this book, the choices of women, and especially mothers, are heavily scrutinized. As we walk through some of your birth options, we want you to know that we are not here to judge you. (Only God and/or Judge Judy can do that.) No two women are the same. Each of us is dealing with our own unique circumstances and preferences. You are not bad or broken for attempting to meet your own physical and emotional needs. Feel free to silence your haters by saying any or all of the following:

"My body, my rules."

"This is not your life."

"What the fuck is your problem?"

"You seem jealous."

"This seems like it's more your issue than mine."

"Seriously, go away."

Your partner should also support and defend your birth choices against anyone who is bothering you, particularly members of their family. This is good practice as you learn to become a stable family unit who sets firm boundaries together. It's important to present a united front.

However your baby is born—you'll have a baby now! And more than that, your pregnancy is finally over! Don't get too down about your decisions or unexpected outcomes. You're doing your best, and you are a champion!

HOW MUCH *SHOULD* YOU DRUG?

One of the first questions you'll ask yourself is whether you'd like your birth to be medicated or unmedicated. There are no easy answers to this question and no one-size-fits-all solution. Here are some questions to ask yourself:

"How high is my pain tolerance?"

How well do you generally deal with pain? For example, stomach pain, menstrual cramps, or being slowly tortured by the gods of creation. If the answer is "not well at all" and you generally sprint toward Tylenol, wine, or any numbing agent you can get your hands on, you may be setting yourself up for failure by attempting an unmedicated labor. Don't get us wrong: you're allowed to do this any way you want to. We just want to be clear—this will likely be the most prolonged "discomfort"* you have ever or will ever experience (unless you've been trapped under a train for several hours). But remember—women have labored without pain meds since the beginning of time—you can do this! But also, you don't have to.

"How sensitive am I to drugs?"

Are you a "lightweight" or someone who is affected differently by certain medications than other people? Then you may want to avoid certain drugs or ask your doctor or anesthesiologist to start you off with the smallest dose possible so you can monitor your

. . . .
* Blinding, unremitting pain

reaction. If you're one of those rare individuals for whom morphine actually *increases* pain, you'll want to make sure the entire hospital knows about it.

"What birth outcome gives me the most anxiety?"

Some would do anything to avoid a C-section.[*] Others are less bothered by surgery or simply need a swift end to a high-risk pregnancy or a difficult birth. Some women are genuinely chill about getting the baby out whatever way necessary. In any case, you're entitled to your own anxieties—as irrational as they may be, you're the one who has to deal with the emotional fallout. Are there incidents in your past that give you specific anxieties about birth? Victims of rape or abuse sometimes find the experience of childbirth especially triggering and may want to make certain preparations to limit the emotional effects. Those sensitive to their surroundings may want to dim the lights or limit the amount of people in the room. If you've been condescended to by male doctors, you may choose to hire a female ob-gyn or midwife. Childbirth is incredibly vulnerable, so arrange whatever assurances you feel you need. We can't promise they'll all go as planned, but you're entitled to your #birthgoalz.

"What are the risks to me and the baby?"

We don't mean to worry you. But we do wish women were given more information. Too often medical options are presented to women without mention of the risks involved. Did you know epidurals occasionally cause an incredibly painful spinal headache, which can last for weeks? It's rare but something you'll definitely wish someone had mentioned in the event it happens to you. Don't go down a rabbit hole of mommy message board conspiracy theories, but do ask questions, do some research, and be your own advocate. And don't ever let a medical professional make you feel guilty for being concerned for your own well-being.

"Which options will be available to me?"

If you're planning a home birth, it's likely that your midwife won't keep many pain-relieving drugs on hand. If you labor at home, there will be no drugs until you get to the hospital. Some hospitals and birthing centers will have a shower or birthing pool. If you're doing a home birth, you can rent a pool. Discuss your options in advance with your provider to see what will be possible.

- - - - - - - - -

[*] While C-sections often save lives, 32 percent of American women undergo them, a rate that falls well above the 10 to 15 percent recommended by the World Health Organization. This means that some women are undergoing major surgery unnecessarily.

Ways Your Birth Plan Might All Go to Hell Anyway

It's good to have realistic expectations so that unfavorable outcomes have less emotional impact. There are many unpredictable factors that can throw off your game plan but can still result in a healthy mother and baby. Know that it will not be the end of the world even if . . .

* you have an unplanned C-section.

* they say it's too late for the epidural when you get to the hospital.

* your anesthesiologist is unavailable at the time you want them to perform the epidural.

* you wanted to labor without painkillers and/or Pitocin, but after hours and hours you need some help.

* you wanted to labor without painkillers, but the pain is so much more than you imagined.

* your epidural doesn't "work."*

* you wanted to birth at the hospital surrounded by medical professionals, but the baby comes out of you before you get there.

* you wanted to labor at home without a needle in your arm, but your water breaks and you need to head to the hospital so you can be monitored and avoid infection.

* you wanted the labor to last about ten minutes and be completely pain-free, but life just didn't work out that way.

. . . .
" Seriously, WTF?

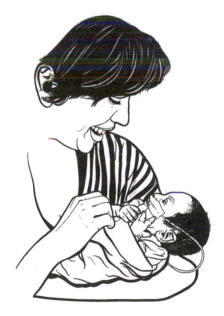

HOME BIRTH: SO YOU'VE DECIDED TO SHIT IN A POOL

When it comes to childbirth, few topics garner more intense opinions on both sides than home birth. We will not be arguing the safety or validity of home birth as a practice, because there is an abundance of information written by well-qualified individuals to guide your decision-making process. Instead, we offer the *very* oversimplified infographic on the next page.

Wondering how to best prepare for the unique and powerful experience of shitting in a small pool in your living room, as several people watch expectantly? Here we go!

SAFETY FIRST!

Right off the bat, there are several easy ways to make your home birth safer:

- Hire a well-qualified midwife (See "A Quick Note on Midwives: CNM and CM versus CPM," on page 27) who ideally has hospital privileges.

- Consider having a backup ob-gyn, just in case.

- Share any unusual medical issues during your pregnancy with your midwife immediately and know what high-risk indicators to look out for toward the end of pregnancy.

- Be flexible and willing to change the plan. An uneventful home birth is the goal, but complications can and do arise, and staying flexible means staying safe.

A FEW UNIQUE BENEFITS OF HOME BIRTH

No Terrible Car Ride to the Hospital/Birth Center

Many women having hospital births try to labor at home for as long as possible. This helps to ensure that they won't be sent home or pressured into interventions that they don't want. If the idea of riding in a moving vehicle during labor sounds like fresh hell, a home birth is a great way to avoid that. If you want a home birth but the car ride sounds fun, go for it, you crazy bitch!

The Freedom

In your own house, you're the boss. You can eat and drink when you want to, yell creative obscenities without offending anyone, get in and out of the shower twenty-five times, and pace around in the nude. You won't be hooked

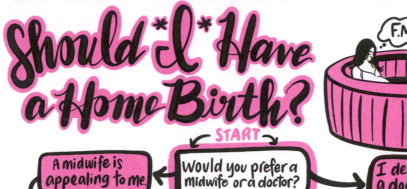

Should *I* Have a Home Birth?

F.M.L.

START

Would you prefer a midwife or a doctor?

A midwife is appealing to me. → **NOICE!** Is your pregnancy low-risk?

I definitely want a doctor to deliver my baby.

NO. High-risk pregnancies should be overseen by a physician.

Yep.

Would you like to try for an unmedicated birth?

Hell No. Pain meds must be administered in a medical setting.

YES.

Cool, so you're kind of a hippie?

I mean, I have an essential oil diffuser, so...yes?

No?

Would you like to be?

Yeah. Strong Start!

No.

Do you have another reason for wanting to do it at home?

Cool cool, does your insurance cover home birth?

Bummer. The U.S. medical system is broken AF and we're sorry. Many women have success appealing this decision, but if not... No.

$ Yeah, girl! $

Huh?

UGH, No.

Can you afford it without adding a ton of stress?

YES.

Find yourself a good witch; you're about to shit in a pool, bitch!

Call and find out! Financial planning for medical bills reduces postpartum stress!

Hospital birth is a great choice for you.

up to a lot of machines or IVs, and so it will be easier to tune in to your body and move in the ways it's asking you to, which will move the baby down, making labor shorter and "easier."

Attentive Care

What you lack in hospital amenities, you may make up for in the one-on-one attention of your home-birth midwife. At home, your midwife has one client: you. She's yours to banish to the living room if you just want to moan alone in bed for a while, and she'll hold your hand through transition, if that's what you end up wanting.

The Comforts of Home

Birthing at home affords you more privacy than in the hospital. Your level of relaxation can help to speed along labor, and some women find they do best with less outside distraction. Also, when it's all over, your midwife/witch will cast her final spell, cleaning up and leaving your home with no evidence of the insane thing that just happened there. You'll go to sleep in your own bed and get a much better night's sleep than you would in a hospital, where nurses are required to do frequent and torturous check-ins with you and your baby.

Postpartum Care

One of the best potential benefits of delivering under the care of a midwife is the level of care you'll receive immediately postpartum. Home-birth midwives will typically visit you and your baby within the first twenty-four hours after birth and will come and/or call you frequently in the first few weeks. She'll help you with breastfeeding, pain management, and check in on your mental health, too. "Midwife" literally translates to "with woman," and she will be. And it will help.

RISKS OF HOME BIRTH

The vast majority of women who give birth at home with a well-qualified midwife do so without complication. However, there is, of course, some risk involved in choosing to deliver outside a hospital setting, and this is something that your midwife should discuss with you at length before you agree to work together. If she doesn't, find another practitioner; a very important part of a midwife's role is to prevent, diagnose, and manage complications to keep you safe, and this means being up front about risk and having a solid safety plan in place. A good midwife has very firm standards about safety and can see an emergency situation coming in plenty of time to prevent it from becoming dangerous. Ask your midwife these questions so you know how she'd deal with a risky situation and you feel comfortable you can trust her.

"What if you're delivering another baby when I go into labor?"

In a hospital setting, if your doctor is delivering another baby, they give you another doctor. What's the plan if this happens at home? Ask her how many clients she has due to deliver in the same month, whether she partners with another midwife for these situations, and if you can meet with that midwife. Most home-birth midwives are very good about stacking their roster and preventing this situation, but remember: due dates are only estimates.

"What if I decide I want pain meds?"

If you're a first-time mom, it can be a little scary to take the leap of faith necessary to have a home birth and forego drugs completely, because what if the pain is just too much? Ask your midwife if she has experience with this scenario (uh, she has, most home births include a brief period of "No, I can't do this; take me to the hospital!"— usually during transition) and what her strategy is for calming you down in those moments.

"What if I need to go to the hospital?"

If you or your baby are in distress, you will need to transfer to a hospital, and this takes time. Ask her under what conditions she requires transfer to a hospital and how you would get there.

"What if I hemorrhage?"

Statistically speaking, postpartum hemorrhage is much less likely after a home birth, as risk of blood loss rises with interventions, but it is still possible. Most issues with bleeding are apparent early and require transfer to a hospital, but in the event that you are losing too much blood at home, what is the plan? Most midwives practice uterine massage to expel any clots after birth, and they also bring the same drugs used to control bleeding in a hospital setting to your birth. You can request that your midwife leave you with a dose of misoprostol at the end of your birth, which can be placed in the cheek to contract the uterus and slow postpartum bleeding in an emergency.

The midwife you want has quick and authoritative answers that address all these risks and any other concerns you may have. Home birth is safe when practiced safely, and you and your baby deserve a safe, happy start.

HOW TO GET READY

Setup for One-Floor Livin'

If your home has more than one floor, you'll want to set up your birthing area on the floor where your bedroom is so that you can easily get in bed with your baby when it's all over and avoid climbing stairs, which increases bleeding.

Gather Your Birth Supplies

Several months before your due date (or your "safe to birth at home" date, which is typically a few weeks before your actual due date and determined by your midwife), you will be given a long list of supplies you'll need to purchase to safely birth at home. The list will vary depending on your provider but may include medical supplies, cleaning products, dog pee pads to bleed onto, plastic mattress covers to go under your sheets, newborn care items, and postpartum supplies for you. All sterile supplies should be kept sealed in their original packaging until their use. You'll need birth linens and other supplies, and baskets. Lots of baskets. Baskets say, "I'm ready to be a mom, because I am very domestic." Fact: the more baskets you have, the better you are at mothering.

The Pool

You're a smart gal, so you probably already figured out that your birth pool will need water. This means that you'll need to measure how far away the pool will be from the nearest bathroom or kitchen sink. Purchase a drinking water hose (so it's lead-free) that's a bit longer than you need, and a hose adapter for your faucet. Ask your witch/midwife how she prefers to empty the pool afterward; some use a fountain pump, and others choose to bail buckets of the bloody water out your front windows, to deter nosy neighbors. Put a tarp under your pool in case anything leaks and so you don't drip bloody water all over your carpet. If you rent a birth pool, purchase a pool liner to protect yourself and the next mom who uses it. Midwives will also sometimes ask you to buy one of those little nets for fish tanks—this is so that they can scoop your turd out of the pool if you accidentally let loose. Are you getting excited about home birth?!

HOME-BIRTH
SUPPLY LIST—ADDENDUM

Here are some "important" items that your midwife may forget to mention:

A Freezer Full of Ice

When nausea hits you hard, you will not want to drink the lukewarm water that your partner is trying to shove in your face between contractions, and if he even mentions the idea of leaving to buy ice, he will not make it out of this shit-show alive. Fill the freezer with ice before go-time, but leave room for the . . .

Frozen Wet Washcloths with Lavender Oil

These are for sniffing and rubbing on your face and neck; they will help you find your chill.

Megaphone

If you can't sleep, why should anyone be able to? Make the whole neighborhood feel your labor "surges" by moaning and groaning di-rectly into a megaphone. You are a powerful goddess, and you will not be ignored.

Sign for Your Front Door

The last thing you need during labor is a police officer showing up to investigate "a disturbance" because you're screaming your head off in the shower. The sign can be a simple "Labor in Progress—Do Not Disturb!" or a playfully menacing riddle, like: "What has two arms when it rings the doorbell and no arms when the door opens? You, if you disturb the laboring woman behind this door!"

If you want to let neighbors know in advance, slip a quick note under their door when you're sure they're not home, or in-person if they're not jerks. If both of these things sound like extroverted torture, just hang a sign on your door and hope for the best. If you think your annoying neighbors or co-op board would have some kind of opposition to you birthing at home, you may want to imply that you're just laboring at home for a while (as many women do) *before* heading to the hospital. You don't owe anyone an explanation, especially the cranky old man who is always accusing you of stealing his mail.

Comfortable Clothing to Rip Off in a Panic

Midwives say they are often able to judge a laboring woman on her progress based on how naked she is, because birth turns us into weird wild animals who suddenly can't stand the feeling of the strappy yoga bra we planned to birth in. Make sure your labor outfit includes lots of clothing that's easy to rip and tear at; you'll almost definitely be completely naked by the time it's over.

Paper and Pen

There is comedy in pain, and one day you'll treasure the tiny scrap of paper where your husband recorded the moment you growled, "STOMP ME OUT LIKE A CAMPFIRE! END ME!"[*]

Encouraging Signage to Snarl At

During the transition stage of labor, it is very common for a woman to say, "Fuck this, I can't do this!" What better place to have that powerful and fleeting moment of existential self-doubt than directly beneath a large hand-lettered sign that reads, "I can do this"? Make it easy to rip.

Yoga or Peanut Ball

Laboring on one of these is a great way to move your baby down faster and "more comfortably" LOL.

. . . .
[*] Attributed to Jackie Ann Ruiz—May 14, 2014

Hospital Bag

Pack one, just in case (see pages 117–119).

. . . .

~~Some~~ People will judge you for having a home birth. Some will congratulate you for "doing it the right way"; ewww, please correct them. There is no right way to give birth; all childbirth is "natural," and birthing at home is not a badge of honor. Other people will judge you for "putting yourself and your baby at risk," and these people can fuck right off too. You do not need to justify your choices to anyone, including family. This is the beginning of a long road where you will be asked to perform motherhood to other people's standards; so come out swingin' and shut that shit right down. You got this, hippie!

WHEN YOU NEED ALL THE DRUGS

Do you want all the drugs? Just a taste? This section is a guide to some of the drugs that you might want/scream for during labor. While there is a risk of side effects with almost any medication, that doesn't mean you shouldn't take something to help you get through the most torturous moment of your life in order to deliver your baby safely. You do, however, deserve to know what you're getting into before someone sticks you with a needle and says, "Don't worry, honey, this is just a little something to calm you down," like it's the Victorian age. It's not the days of twilight sleep,* and you're a literate woman who deserves some say in her medical care.

DRUGS FOR WHEN YOU WANT THE PAIN TO START

Maybe your membranes ruptured (your water broke) but you're not going into labor. Or maybe your labor keeps stopping and starting. Or maybe you're a week past your due date and want to get this show on the road. Uterotonics are drugs that induce labor, meaning they stimulate uterine contractions. These are the drugs that press play on pushing a baby out.

Prostaglandin Induction—Cervidil and Cytotec (Misoprostol)

Prostaglandin induction is used to ripen the cervix before your contractions have begun. It is often followed by other induction medications, which will help to start or strengthen contractions. Cervidil is a vaginal insert (sort of like a tampon), and Cytotec is a pill (usually administered vaginally). Prostaglandins carry a risk for uterine rupture, but it is a far smaller risk than sensational coverage might have you believe. The risk is much higher in women attempting VBAC (vaginal birth after cesarean delivery); therefore it is generally not prescribed to women who have previously undergone cesareans.

Oxytocin (Pitocin)

Oxytocin is a naturally occurring hormone in your body, responsible for, among other things, inducing labor. Oxytocin is confus-

---

* "Twilight sleep" was a mixture of heavy drugs often given to laboring women in the early to mid-twentieth century that would leave them with no memory of their labor and sometimes serious side effects.

DRUGS!

For when you say

WHAT?

HOW?

EPIDURAL

A catheter (tube) is inserted into your spine with a needle to administer IV fluids. The area is numbed first with another needle, which feels like a bee sting. You'll need to keep VERY still while it's being placed—even if you're having a contraction—which is...insane. It lasts longer than a spinal, but takes longer to kick in.

In a standard epidural, the catheter is placed just outside the spinal fluid, and contains local anesthetics which make your lower body feel fairly numb + dead. Some women love this, while others find it dis-orienting. Moving your body will probably require assistance.

A walking epidural goes directly into the spinal fluid + is a combo of anesthetic, narcotic and epinephrine. You will still have some sensation in your lower body, which allows for easier move-ment, and may help labor progress. Despite the name, you will most likely not be able to "walk."

SPINAL BLOCK

Very similar to epidural, except instead of a catheter drugs are delivered via a one-time spinal injection, which provides pain relief for around 2 hours.

Usually only used for planned C-Sections, and sometimes vaginal births for women who have already had a child, where labor is moving quickly and there's not enough time for an epidural to take effect.

NO NO NO NOoooo!! MAKE IT STOP!

POSSIBLE SIDE EFFECTS!

- Low blood pressure
- Loss of bladder control
- Itchy skin
- Nausea
- Slow breathing
- Spinal headache (1/100)
- Nerve damage (RARE)
- Epidural just flat out not working for some goddess-forsaken reason...?

HOT TIPS!

- Find out your hospital's policy on eating, drinking, and moving around once you've had the epidural.

- There may be time in your labor to try an analgesic and epidural if one or the other is not to your liking.

- Drugs can be turned down later if you want more sensation or to be more alert when the baby arrives, but it may take time for the epidural to wear off.

- Since the drugs are roughly the same, side effects are similar to those mentioned for epidurals + analgesics.

- In the event of an emergency C-section, you may have a combo spinal + epidural, which combines the immediate relief of a spinal and the sweet, sweet staying power of an epidural.

more →

HOW?

WHAT?

ANALGESICS

Opiates are administered through a one-time injection in your spine, an IV in your hand or arm, or a PCA pump, where you get to control the dose yourself like a greedy-ass dope fiend.

Unlike an epidural, analgesics won't fully numb your pain; they take the edge off. These meds may make you feel sleepy and relaxed, or they may make you feel disoriented and dizzy. Some women report feeling "high as balls," while others may report feeling "way too high."

NITROUS, A.K.A. "LAUGHING GAS," A.K.A. "Remember whip its?!"

Gas is administered via a breathing mask that you are able to control yourself.

Not as strong as other analgesics. You may still feel labor pain but will likely perceive it as less intense. Nitrous oxide does not affect your body's release of oxytocin, the progress of your labor, or the alertness of your baby.

DRUGS!

POSSIBLE SIDE EFFECTS!

HOT TIPS!

- Nausea
- Vomiting
- Breathing problems
- Feeling really, really fucking itchy, like a street addict in an overacted 80s movie.
- Opiates cross the placenta, so they can have negative effects on your baby's breathing, central nervous system, neurological behavior, ability to breastfeed early on, and ability to regulate body temperature.

- Analgesics can also be turned down later in your labor and will wear off more quickly than epidural.

- Sleepiness
- Nausea
- Vomiting
- Nitrous can deplete your body's B12 vitamins and should not be used if your levels are low. Ask to have your levels checked, if you plan to use it.

- Use of this low-risk and effective drug is still rare in the U.S., so find out if it's available to you. If it isn't, then complain. #BETHECHANGE

ingly *also* the name of the synthetic drug version of that hormone. Pitocin is the brand name of that drug. Therefore Pitocin and oxytocin are the same thing, sometimes. Got it? Your health-care provider may prescribe this drug to induce or increase the strength of contractions. They may also administer Pitocin after you deliver in order to shrink the uterus more quickly, which controls bleeding and helps you expel the placenta. Yep, just another weird thing you have to look forward to!

It's debatable whether Pitocin and other induction methods cause contractions to be more painful. They do bring on stronger contractions more quickly, which are naturally going to be the most painful part of labor. But outside of having a cesarean, these stronger contractions are something you will need to experience in order for your baby to be born. So, *shrug emoji.*

Other Drugs

Other drugs you may need before or after the birth of your baby include:

- Drugs to stop preterm labor
- Antibiotics to prevent infection, particularly if you are strep B positive
- Drugs to slow rapid labor, such as magnesium, which can make you feel sleepy AF
- Drugs to treat preeclampsia, which include the aforementioned sleep-inducing magnesium
- Drugs to slow bleeding after delivery
- Drugs to calm you down or help you sleep

These are just some of the most common medications administered during labor. We are not doctors and cannot predict how your body will be affected by specific medications. We wish you the best and hope you feel confident and supported in your decisions. Talk to your provider about any and all concerns.

TRYING TO STAY OFF THE DRUGS

Whether you're just trying to get through the hours before you're admitted to the hospital, or you labor entirely unmedicated, having some tips in your back pocket for more "natural" pain relief isn't a bad idea. Tell your provider if you're going to attempt an unmedicated birth. It's possible they'll still offer you drugs during labor, but if you're on the same page, they'll hopefully do so less frequently or only when medically necessary.

We think every woman has a right to labor without drugs, but we also concede that there are situations when doing so would be dangerous or traumatic for the baby and/or mother. Having an unmedicated birth does not make you better than other moms, but if it's the preferred and safe decision for you—go for it. And if you change your mind at any time, for any reason, there's no shame in that.

NATURAL WAYS TO GET THINGS GOING

If you want your labor to get going, there are some drug-free methods that might help. Note that any methods that involving insert-ing something into the vagina are inadvisable once your membranes have ruptured, since that could introduce bacteria and cause infection.

Remember: Never attempt to induce labor until you are cleared by your health-care provider to do so.

Castor oil: Castor oil is a laxative that causes your bowels to contract, which often in turn stimulates your uterus to contract. Basically you're giving yourself a ton of gas pain that leads right into labor pain. On the plus side, you probably won't poop later in labor, because you'll already have shit all your brains out. Like all natural induction methods, this will probably only lead to labor if your body is already somewhat ready for it.

Castor oil is very difficult to drink; not because it tastes particularly bad but because it is very slippery and feels sort of like ingesting an anti-frizz hair product. Your body will gag and protest, so there are many different methods of tricking your body into not puking it up. Some people prefer to just take it as a shot and follow with a chaser of orange juice, while others mix the two together and chug. Some prefer to make the world's worst omelet, and still others swear by the world's worst root beer float. Whatever method you choose, consult with your health-care professional beforehand.

Acupuncture: Acupuncture is a practice from traditional Chinese medicine that involves inserting very tiny needles into specific points on your body. A recent study[1] shows that acupuncture, performed on women after their membranes have ruptured, may induce cervical ripening but does not reduce the need for Pitocin or other induction. Potential side effects are minor. Basically, if you're into it, it might be worth a try, but you'll never really know how much it helped, if at all.

Pressure-point stimulation: Hate needles? Many of the acupuncture points used to induce labor can also be massaged, which means you can do it at home, which means you don't have to put on pants! Gently massage these points (alternating sides of your body between rounds) by simply applying moderate pressure or rubbing in small circles for a few minutes, and if you start to feel uterine contractions, that might be a good spot for you to continue to work on. Take breaks and breathe deeply during the contractions to relax and encourage your body to keep it going, and wait a few minutes before massaging again. The next page offers a few spots to try.

Stripping membranes, a.k.a. membrane sweeping: In order to strip the membranes, a doctor or midwife will insert their gloved finger into the cervix and gently separate the uterine sac from the side of the uterus. This releases hormones that can trigger contractions. This can be *very* uncomfortable and may cause cramping and spotting, but early labor also causes those things, so if you're tired of waiting, do it!

Sex: It probably won't instantly induce labor, but sex can trigger the release of oxytocin, which helps contractions. Orgasms can stimulate your uterus into action, and male sperm helps soften the cervix. If the idea of sex is at all appealing to you now, go for it! You'll likely be off sex for at least six weeks postpartum (more if you're as tired as we were) so enjoy it while you still can, if you can even enjoy it now.

Feeling like there's "no room at the inn"? ("The inn" being a playful euphemism for your insides, which cannot comfortably accommodate a penis at the moment.) Reach around that big ol' belly and help yourself, or have your partner use a vibrator on you.

Nipple stimulation: You can twiddle your own nips or have your partner stimu-

Pressure Points

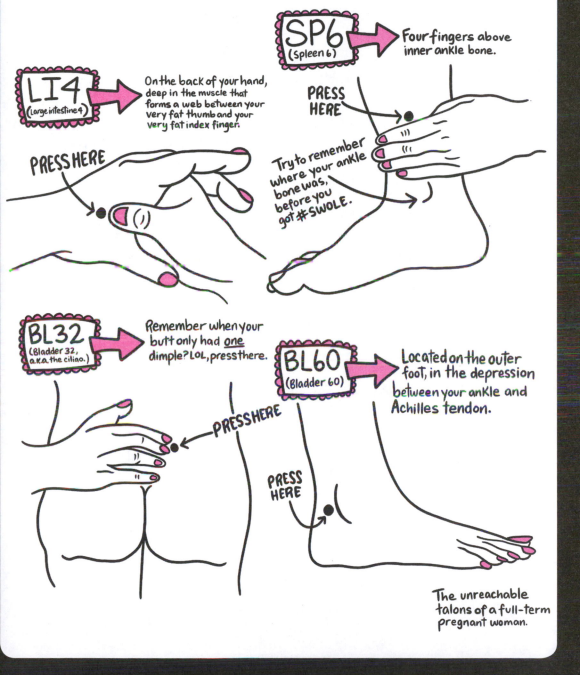

SP6 (Spleen 6) → Four fingers above inner ankle bone.

LI4 (Large intestine 4) → On the back of your hand, deep in the muscle that forms a web between your very fat thumb and your very fat index finger.

PRESS HERE

Try to remember where your ankle bone was, before you got #SWOLE.

PRESS HERE

BL32 (Bladder 32, a.k.a. the ciliao.) → Remember when your butt only had _one_ dimple? LOL, press there.

PRESS HERE

BL60 (Bladder 60) → Located on the outer foot, in the depression between your ankle and Achilles tendon.

PRESS HERE

The unreachable talons of a full-term pregnant woman.

late with their hands or mouth. This only works if it feels good, which will release oxytocin, which can trigger contractions if your body is otherwise ready and just needs to chill out a little. Take breaks from nipple stimulation during contractions, unless your body tells you otherwise. Some advice suggests using a breast pump for nipple stim, but breast pumps are actual torture and no one should have to use them until they *have* to use them.

Eat eggplant, and other probably useless lore: There are too many "surefire" ways to go into labor, we couldn't possibly list them all here (that's what your smartphone is for). In every town in America, there is a restaurant that makes a special eggplant Parmesan that puts women into instant labor. Eat it; food is delicious, and you are very hungry. Some women swear by curb-walking, which is when you walk in the street with one foot up on the curb. Do it: walking is good for you.

Feeling ready: None of these things are going to work all that well if you don't feel ready to go into labor. Our bodies are wise and will try to postpone labor until a woman is calm, safe, and ready. So, if you've got some last-minute task in your head that's nagging you, do it. If someone is around you who makes you feel unsafe, get some help to make them leave. If you're wishing you had gone to get a final pedicure/haircut/sensory-deprivation-tank float, make it happen. Do what makes you feel good, ready, safe, and happy, and your body will get the message.

NONMEDICAL PAIN MANAGEMENT

You'll notice we didn't say pain relief, because if you don't take drugs you're going to be in pain.[*] That doesn't mean there aren't a lot of ways to help manage and decrease your pain though.

Get a Fun Doula

You want a doula who reminds you of your best friend, because you'll feel comfortable being honest about what you want and need from them, allowing you to make the most of your relationship and get the support that you need.[†]

....

[*] Unless you're one of those unicorn women we hear about from time to time. If you are, we maybe don't want to hear about it.

[†] Learn more about doulas in "Your Live Studio Audience," page 114.

Find Water

Laboring in a birth tub or shower can offer some serious pain relief. Floating in water takes a lot of pressure off your belly, and the warm water relaxes your muscles and helps your labor progress. Running warm water on your lower back can be soothing, particularly during early labor at home.

Pay attention to what the water does to your contractions—does it make them weaker or stronger? Once labor gets going, you want to keep it going, so if the water relaxes your body so much that you kind of feel like you're not really in labor anymore, then the water is a resting spot for you. Take a minute to get your strength up, and then get out. Once you stand, your labor is likely to get more intense again. Remember, the more intense it gets, the closer you are to the end.

Use Rebozo Sifting

A rebozo is a long, woven scarf that is traditionally used by Mexican women but is gaining popularity in the American birth community. Mexican women use the scarf for many things throughout their lives: wrapped around a pregnant belly for support, later carrying the baby on the chest or back, and as a pain-relief tool in labor with a process known as "sifting."

It's a good idea to watch some instructional videos and get plenty of practice before trying to incorporate this into your labor. Or have someone already practiced, like your doula, do it for you.

Sifting throughout your pregnancy stimulates the parasympathetic nervous system, making you feel calmer and more relaxed; so if you enjoy it, practice often. You may find that you like the sensation, or you may feel like you're trapped inside one of those fat-vibrating machines from the 1950s. It's good to know these things beforehand. Do not use a rebozo if there is threat of a miscarriage, and ask your health-care provider before doing any new stuff to your body.

If you choose to purchase a traditional rebozo, snag one from a respectful fair-trade company that is owned by Mexican women, since the rebozo is traditionally made by women for women, and that's dope.

To use it, wrap the scarf over your belly and have a helper hold the ends as you kneel and lean onto a birth ball or chair, draping your arms and settling into a relaxed pose. Use pillows to support your knees and anywhere else that helps you get comfortable.

Your helper should stand behind you with slightly bent knees, holding the ends of the rebozo like the reins of a horse, with straight wrists and strong arms. As your helper slowly lifts your belly and relieves pressure and weight from your spine, you might make sex noises, and this is okay, because you are a sexy, sexy beast and also it feels very good. Slow, short movements from your helper's wrists will vibrate your belly, releasing tension and encouraging your body to relax and make room for your baby to come down. Communicate with your helper about what speed and pressure feels best, and stop when it stops helping.

Get a Counterpressure Massage

This isn't massage so much as someone pushing on you. Your doula (or whoever is assisting you, if they've been shown how) can press firmly onto your lower back or squeeze your hips together to alleviate some of the back pain, especially if you're having back labor.

Walk, Rock, and Shake Your Booty

Moving around and finding the right position can vastly increase your comfort and help the baby to move downward. Assuming you're not strapped to a monitor or otherwise restricted, you should try to move around, if only as a distraction. You can pace the halls, swing your hips from side to side, or do a lot of cat-cow poses in bed. Some women like to hang from straps, which can be found in some birth centers. If you don't have something to hang on, use your partner. Find positions that feel right for you. And if things are stalling out, force yourself to move even if it feels like the worst thing on earth. Sometimes pain is increased by the poor position of the baby, and the best way to alleviate that pain is to shake the baby loose from whatever corner they've wedged themselves into.*

Use Birthing or Peanut Balls

An inflatable yoga or peanut ball can be helpful for rocking your hips or positioning your legs comfortably. Some doulas and midwives will bring them along. Someone will have to sterilize this thing later when it's covered in your fluids, but that's all part of the magic of life.

Use Visualization and Meditation

Visualizations and other methods can help keep you calm and focused. Depending on how your labor is going, you may find that this is easier said than done. While it may not help during the blinding pain of transition, it might relax you in early labor, when you're feeling the jitters and your body hasn't completely taken over.

. . . .
* For more position inspo, see "The Weirdness of Labor," page 130.

Moan Like a Large Mammal

One of the most baffling things about labor is the idea that you must "relax into the pain." Intellectually this sentence makes almost zero sense; how could anyone relax while in that much physical discomfort, when the normal instinct is to tighten and contract against painful feelings? Channeling your animal self, that's how.

Most of us grew up watching movies and TV that portrayed laboring women on their backs, shrieking the high-pitched song of a jungle bird in distress. Since then, we have learned a lot as a culture, including which living things do not give birth and should not be allowed to write about it. Here are two: birds and male writers.

Across the mammalian world, labor sounds pretty much the same: deep, low, and slow moaning; strong exhalations with floppy horse lips; and a lot of deep "AAAAA" and "OOOO" sounds. These are the sounds of a relaxed body, the key to a faster and more efficient dilation and birth.

There's science behind this! Low vocalization in your throat focuses the pressure of your pushes onto your diaphragm rather than your throat, making your pushes more effective. The lower the sound, the wider your throat is opening as you make it, which allows for deeper breathing and relaxed shoulders. The widened mouth position required to sound like a bored demon also relaxes the powerful muscles of your face and jaw, releasing tension.

In Ina May Gaskin's "Sphincter Law" (hahahahahahaha okay, no, stop, this is a real thing) she explains that there is a direct correlation between your mouth and your cervix, vagina, and sphincter. When your mouth and jaw are relaxed, your bottom will be more relaxed, allowing your baby to move down and GTFO of your body ASAP.

Since we tend to keep a lot of tension in our facial muscles, it can take some practice to fully understand what it feels like to relax your face. Practice with a simple exercise called progressive muscle relaxation. This technique involves taking a deep, relaxing breath and then tensing a muscle group to maximum intensity and holding for several seconds before releasing on your exhale. Do this several times; it's normal to feel a warm or tingling sensation as your body sends blood to your muscles to help them relax.

Understanding this feeling will help you be aware of your facial tension during labor and allow you to relax your muscles fully during a contraction. Bonus: you can use this technique to relax any muscle in your body, and if you do it in public, no one will try to talk to you or touch your belly bump because you will look dangerously unstable.

Use Essential Oils

We know, that anti-vax woman you went to middle school with keeps inviting you to buy essential oils and ugly leggings, so it sort of feels like it's all bullshit. Seriously, don't buy those leggings, but essential oils are an ancient idea backed by research,[2] which confirms their effectiveness in reducing labor anxiety, fear, and sometimes even pain.

Essential oils are very concentrated, and so most should *never* be applied directly to skin. Use a carrier oil such as coconut, grapeseed, or sweet almond oil and follow the directions on the bottle. Once diluted, the oil can be applied to the skin during massage or dabbed onto your pressure points. Don't want to be touched? Us either: add the undiluted oil to a diffuser while growling, "I NEED SOME SPACE," and sniff that shit instead.

Lavender: There's a reason why this scent is so popular with women; it's calming AF, and Mama is *stressed*. Cool your jets with a few sniffs of this potent purple flower during pregnancy, labor, or for postpartum anxiety and sleep issues.

Frankincense: While there's actually no such thing as a wise man, the men who brought this shit to a postpartum Mary knew a thing or two. Like lavender, it is calming and can also be rubbed into areas of tension during labor to relieve pain. Vaginal tears may heal more quickly when treated with frankincense, too!

Myrrh: Labor stalling out? Put a few drops of myrrh oil on a washcloth and sniff; it may help contractions get stronger. It's also a good noise to make in labor; let's try it now: "MYRRRRH." You sound silly.

Peppermint or spearmint: A drop of mint oil directly on your tongue can increase energy during the marathon stage of labor and can help fight nausea during pregnancy and labor. A few drops on a wet washcloth applied to the skin can cool down an overheating body, and mixed with a carrier oil can be massaged into sore muscles to relieve aches and pains. Some women with breech babies have even had success turning them by rubbing some peppermint oil onto the tops of their bellies, because while babies may seem to be 100 percent pure love, they're all born into this world with an intense hatred for only one thing: mint. An unexpected challenge of late pregnancy and labor can be emptying your bladder. If you have to pee and can't, sit on the toilet and sniff some peppermint oil while taking nice, slow deep breaths—it works!

Clary sage: *Note: may induce labor, so do not use during pregnancy, and get the okay from your health-care provider before using.*

Clary sage can help some women start or ramp up their contractions, if their body is ready. As a massage oil, it can also be used for pain relief and relaxation, and it smells really good.

Once your baby is born, you should carefully research any oils you keep near them, especially if you're applying it to a part of your or their body where they might touch and/or ingest it. Babies should never take essential oils orally, though some can be safely rubbed on their bellies or other body parts. Talk to your health-care provider, because even just diffusing certain oils around infants can be harmful.

WHEN NONE OF THIS SHIT IS ENOUGH

No matter what kind of birth you planned to have, remember that there is *zero* shame in needing medication to relieve your pain, especially if it gets so intense that you feel like you can't go on. Every labor is different, and every birth story is a story of triumph and warrior badassery. No matter how this all turns out, you fucking *Did. It.* Go you.

LET'S TALK ABOUT C-SECTIONS

C-sections happen for any number of reasons, none of which are your "fault." There is nothing to gain in feeling shame over any measure you take to ensure the safety of yourself or your baby. It may not be your ideal birth scenario, but it's sometimes helpful to know what a C-section involves, so that should you experience one, it's not as scary. While there is risk associated with any surgery, C-sections are generally considered safe. C-sections fall into two camps: emergency C-sections and planned C-sections.

EMERGENCY CESAREAN SECTION

Emergency C-sections can happen for a variety of reasons when you are planning to attempt a vaginal birth—your labor stalls for too long, the baby is in distress, or you are in distress. Mothers will often be given an epidural or spinal block if there is time so that they can stay awake during the procedure. If the baby needs to be born quickly, anesthesia will be administered to put you to sleep. If you are awake, you shouldn't feel any pain, but you will feel a tugging sensation as they are pulling the baby out of you. There is often a curtain between you and your belly, and your arms may be strapped down. While that might sound scary and intense, the operating table is pretty thin so that doctors can reach across your body, and being strapped down while heavily drugged on a tiny table is sort of reassuring in the moment.

TAP BLOCK

An alternative to an epidural or spinal, a TAP block is a type of anesthetic injected locally into your abdominal muscles to numb the nerves. The pain relief lasts forty to seventy-two hours, meaning C-section moms are able to take fewer other drugs and deal with fewer side effects of those drugs as they are meeting their baby. This is a relatively new procedure in birth, so if you are planning a C-section, you may want to ask your provider about it.

If you were not planning to have a C-section, it's okay to feel sad, disappointed, or traumatized; this hiccup in the plan is not the end of the world, but it's okay to feel that way for a bit. After you feel your feelings, try to focus on the marvel of modern medicine that allowed your baby's safe arrival into your arms, and squeeze them tight. For C-section recovery, see page 152.

PLANNED CESAREAN SECTION

There are many reasons your doctor may schedule a C-section, including health issues, carrying multiples, previous C-section, or your preference for one. Mothers with planned cesareans have the benefit of knowing what's up, and it's usually calmer than an unexpected C-section. Planned C-sections will be scheduled, so you'll know your baby's birthday in advance and may even have some say in deciding it, which is cool! The anticipation is often worse than the C-section itself, so don't worry! Here are some tips if you have the luxury of planning:

- **Ask about the hospital's policy on eating or drinking before the procedure.** You normally can't eat for eight hours prior, but they may let you sneak some water in there if it's not too close to go time.

- **Try to bring as little as possible.** You'll have to declare all items as if you're entering prison, so you may not feel like listing out every little thing. Don't worry, they'll have everything you need, including what you'll wear as you recover.

- **Ask your doctor to check if you have diastasis recti* while they're in there.** They might be able to stitch it back together a bit, which will aid recovery. This is a cool benefit of a C-section!

- **Prepare for a lot of waiting.** Once admitted, you'll be taken to a prep room, where you'll change into your gown, get your vitals taken, get an IV, and meet with the anesthesiologist, who will go over what's about to happen. Your partner or support person may have to wait outside the operating room while you're prepped. After that they can usually come in to hold your hand.

- **If you can't hold the baby right away, have your partner do skin-to-skin.†** One benefit of being out of commission is that your partner gets to bond with the baby right away. You'll probably have to wait awhile as they take out your placenta and stitch you up.

* Diastasis recti is when your abdominal muscles separate. For more on this, see page 198.

† For more on skin-to-skin, see page 138.

- **Then get ready for more waiting/ moving/being bothered.** After surgery you'll be moved to a recovery room where they'll monitor you while the anesthesia wears off. You may still feel a bit weird and woozy, but you'll finally get to spend time with your baby. After about an hour they'll move you to your actual room, where nurses will continue to check frequently. Let them know if you're not getting enough sleep, so they can try to interrupt less often.

- Remind your partner in advance to text your family that everything went okay. This is easy to forget in all the excitement of meeting your baby.

OTHER WEIRD STUFF TO BE PREPARED FOR IN A C-SECTION

- **They'll shave your pubes.** The incision will probably be low on your stomach, which is nice if you still wanna rock a two-piece, but they gotta get those pubes out of the way. Don't feel the need to prepare your pubes. They do this all the time.

- **Assuming you're awake for the procedure, you'll get an epidural, spinal, or TAP block.** The needle or catheter situation can be momentarily weird, but it'll be over quickly (see page 110).

- **They'll insert a catheter into your pee hole.** This is usually done after anesthesia, so you won't feel it. Urine is collected into a bag that nurses will change as needed, and everyone will know exactly how hydrated you are. Post-surgery it may feel irritated or like you need to pee, and it will be one more thing getting in the way of your movement. On the plus side, you don't have to get up to go to the bathroom while you're recovering from surgery.

- **The pain meds might make you shaky or weak afterward.** Sometimes women feel like there is a weight on their lungs, like they can't breathe. Don't worry, you can breathe.

- **There will be a bright light in your face.** This, combined with the curtain separating you from your body, can make you feel a bit like a science experiment. Focus on your support person, who should help keep you calm.

- **You can smell burning skin.** Thankfully you're not feeling this!

- **Doctors will probably be super casual or cheerful.** This is a good thing! They do this all the time.

- **They'll use stitches or staples to put you back together.** They're both easy to take out and probably won't look as bad as you expect once the bandages are removed.

FAMILY-CENTERED C-SECTION

Many doctors now offer "family-centered" cesareans or "gentle" cesareans. This is meant to give more focus to the mother and allow her to be more connected to the birth process. Often the mother can see the baby come out via a clear drape, a window in the curtain, or a mirror. In some cases, the mother's arms are not strapped down, so that she can hold and breastfeed the baby right away. If that is not possible, doctors may still be able to place the baby cheek to cheek with you, which is a great way to connect with your baby for a moment before they start tending to you both. Doctors may even let the umbilical cord pulse for a while before cutting it, so that the baby can receive more of the cord blood. These measures may not be possible in emergency scenarios, but if there's time to discuss, ask your doctor what's possible.

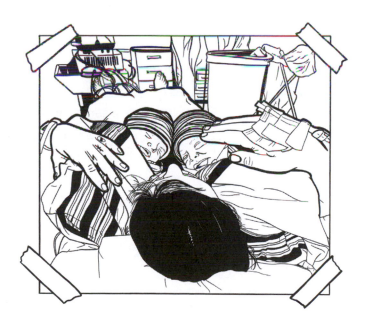

YOUR LIVE STUDIO AUDIENCE

Building your birth team is a crucial step in planning your birth; you want to stack your roster with supportive, strong, loving people who will not hold a grudge when they offer you a washcloth and you shove their hand away. Birth is emotionally intense, and you don't need to worry about anyone else's feelings.

Deciding who can watch you squirm and holler is a personal preference. Some people need their mom or their BFF. Some people want as few people as possible. Sometimes you want a doula who just "gets it." Here are some of your options.

DOCTORS AND NURSES

If you're birthing in the hospital, they actually have, like, a whole setup where doctors and nurses are scheduled to be there and you don't even have to worry about it. Doctors don't normally attend home births, but maybe you have, like, a dermatologist in the family you could invite?

MIDWIFE

If you're birthing at home, a birth center, or somewhere in the woods, you'll want to have a midwife with you.* That YouTube video of a woman birthing unassisted and barefoot on the rocks next to a babbling stream is pretty badass, but please bring a midwife to your stream birth. A seasoned and well-qualified midwife will keep you and your baby safe in the event of a complication and will mostly leave you alone to do yo' thang if everything is proceeding normally.

PARTNER

If you have a partner, you'll probably want them there. Have them watch some birth videos before the big day, so they understand that There Will Be Blood. If your partner is Daniel Day-Lewis, he already knows that, but you should probably ask him to tell you in that voice, just for birth-tub shits and giggles.

SHOULD YOU GET A DOULA?

If you're planning to attempt a drug-free birth, a labor doula can be a great support person during labor. Doulas are trained in pregnancy and labor and are equipped with pain-management strategies that can make a big difference in the length of your labor. Scientific trials have found that doula care im-

* Midwives also sometimes work out of regular hospitals.

proves psychological and physical outcomes for both mother and baby. They are not medical professionals; think of them as wizards. They're exactly like wizards.

A doula will make sure you're drinking enough water and peeing often and changing positions, she will put good-smelling oils on warm washcloths and wipe your face and do counterpressure massage and maybe sift your belly with a rebozo* and lots of things that you will either love or hate, and it won't hurt her feelings when you scream, "No, don't move your hand at all—just press! NO RUBBING!" All of these things will go a long way toward keeping your stamina up in the marathon of labor. Your doula may also talk your partner or support person through some of the ways they can support/rub you, assuming they don't make a regular habit of attending live births.

Your doula is also your personal advocate, the person who will stand up for your birth plan when you can't speak in English anymore because the contractions are coming too fast and someone is trying to change your plan. If your partner or another support person can do this for you, or if the idea of having someone you haven't known for very long in the room while you're nude and yelling a lot makes you feel nervous, or

you just can't bear the cost of yet another baby-related service, maybe you don't want a doula. If the cost is your only hesitation, many hospitals now have volunteer doulas!

FAMILY AND FRIENDS

According to our anecdotal research, some people genuinely like their family and would enjoy having them in the room during such an important life event. Other people may have recently moved five states away to escape their family; it takes all kinds!

When it comes to letting family and friends attend your labor, go with your gut. If they're a calming presence, let them watch your vag expand! If they're pressuring you to let them be there, DO NOT INVITE THEM TO YOUR BIRTH (this includes the hospital waiting room). This is your struggle, your baby, you you you. They have no business there unless you want them. You have no responsibility to let them near you while you recover. Having a baby is hard! Do not let other people make it worse, no matter what they mean to you.

Remember, setting the boundaries you need will allow you to be a calmer, healthier presence for your baby. You have so much on your plate those first few weeks and deserve every concession you can get. Labor is a vul-

---

* See page 105 for more info on rebozos, ya bozo!

nerable time, and you probably want to keep the crowd small and intimate. But reserve the right to change your mind at the last second and decide you need five best friends to feed you Popsicles while you push.

If you're not close with your family but would still like to have "your people" there, inviting a close friend to your birth is a great solution. After reading this, you probably already have the right person in mind.

WHAT OTHER BOOKS MAY TELL YOU
TO PACK IN YOUR HOSPITAL BAG!

The Perfect Playlist

If you're really musically inclined, give it a go, but it's very possible that labor will make you forget that music is even a thing that exists, or you may demand total silence. So don't stress too hard about finding the right tunes; you can always scream, "Hey, Siri, play 'Best of My Love'! *No!* Not the Eagles, the Emotions!" If you do make a mix, make two; one to pump you up and one to chill you out. Your labor will give you strong and unpredictable needs and opinions.

Gifts or Treats for the Hospital Staff

Yes, they do a lot, but it is their job. You are having a baby, that is a *lot*. If doing this makes you feel genuinely good, go for it; we just want you to know that you're not shitty if you *don't* do it.

A Fancy-Pants Camera

Unless this thing comes with its own professional photographer, it's not likely to make it out of your bag. Plus, cell phone cameras take amazing photos now, and you can easily share your first family photos with your loved ones from your hospital bed while you breastfeed and stuff your face like a *victorious queen*.

A Printed Copy of Your Birth Plan

Bring this if your partner is a spaz, but they should really know this info by now. . . . Get it together, Brad!

A Bathing Suit

You want to cover up in the birth tub/ shower? Okay, but in a few hours everyone in the room will be staring directly into your junk, right before they inspect your nipple to show you how to breastfeed. You're basically family now, and it's a naked family! *Only you and your baby are allowed to be nude at your baby's birth!* Aww, twinsies!

Toiletries, Hairbrush, Makeup, Etc.

Sure, you'll want some of this stuff, but we hope you don't feel like you need to "fix your face" after giving birth. If there was ever a time to embrace looking like a hot mess, it is right after you soft-serve a baby out of your body. Hospital bathrooms are very small and don't have a lot of space to put things; don't be a hero.

Slippers or Socks

Okay, these aren't a bad idea, but if you bring your good ones, you might want to burn them after they've touched a hospital floor. The hospital will provide socks, which they will be happy to burn for you when you are discharged. Your insurance will be billed $600 for this service.

Christmas Lights

We get it; mood lighting. Let's do a thought experiment, okay? How do you react when you stub the shit out of your toe? Now imagine stubbing the shit out of your vagina, every two to four minutes for several hours. Now imagine that while this is happening your partner is struggling to untangle Christmas lights, and they do so much as *lightly* sigh in frustration while you're in excruciating pain. Yeah, pack light. Keep it simple.

Something Reassuring, Like a Photo of Someone You Love

Again, if this feels really crucial for you, go for it. If not, leave more space in your bag for other things you'll want, like an entire bag of dark chocolates.*

WHAT YOU ACTUALLY NEED TO BRING

Nail File

Don't bother packing the baby-size nail clippers; those come later. While your perfect angel will likely be born with freakishly long White Walker talons, newborn nails are still weirdly attached to their finger skin, aww! Super . . . cute . . . ? If you try to use clippers you may end up cutting them, and you deserve some postpartum recovery time before your first "I hurt my baby by accident" shame spiral. Some people file the nails down, but lots of us end up chewing them off. Seriously; it's the gentlest way and your animal hormones already make you want to eat your adorable kin, so go with God.

A Change of Clothes

This will be your outfit for the ride home once you ditch the hospital gown. Keep it comfy; keep it loose. You will be exhausted, twelve different kinds of sore, and your belly will still be very big; that shit takes time. Sweatshirts and long-sleeved shirts should zip or button up, so you can get at them boobies.

Snacks

Whether they let you eat during labor, remember that you're in this for the long haul. Think about what you might like to eat when this marathon is finally over. Pack some favorites and consider something high in protein like trail mix or some energy bars, in case the food at the hospital is truly putrid. You'll need to get your energy back up, and if you plan to breastfeed, you've got a lot of milk to make. Ordering delivery to your hospital room is also *more* than okay—you've earned it. Order dessert.

* Do this, either way.

An Outfit for Your Baby

The hospital will provide swaddles and onesies, but once you leave, you're gonna need to put some clothes on that kid. Make sure it's something with legs (not a sleep sack) so you can separate their legs to get them in the car seat. If it's cold out, pack some warm outerwear; newborns have a harder time regulating body temperature, because they are used to being inside you. Don't worry about packing a jacket for your partner; by the time you give birth, he will be used to not being inside you.

A Phone Charger

You're gonna have to text the whole fam about what just went down. Bring a long one in case the outlet is far from the bed.

A Toothbrush

Your mouth will thank you.

Your ID, Insurance Card, and Other Boring Adult Papers

Be prepared to fill out tons of paperwork (a fun thing to do during your baby's first days on earth)! You may be pretty brain-dead and forget your own name, so any relevant info is worth bringing along so you don't have to think too hard after being in labor for what felt like nine years.

Nursing Bra

While you're at the hospital you'll probably let those puppies hang loose, but as you dress for the ride home you will want something soft and comfy that keeps your nips handy. Are you getting that the ability to whip out your tits on the fly is a very large part of early motherhood? Not breastfeeding? No matter; you're still allowed to pull a boob out literally whenever and wherever you want! It's the law, look it up!

A Car Seat

Dear Lord, do not forget this one. They won't let you take your baby home without one. This one may seem obvious, but when you're a human beach ball it becomes pretty damn easy to drop the ball and start forgetting important shit. Car seats and buckles can be tricky, so read reviews and survey your coven to find one that you won't throw into traffic in frustration. Most hospitals can double-check your installation, or you can find a firehouse near you that has a certified car seat technician. Stop by and ogle some firemen while they sexily make sure your baby will ride safe.

Hair Ties

Put a few in every pocket of your bag; this will make it easier for your skittish partner to find when you threaten to shave your own head if someone doesn't hand you one. Immediately.

WAITING IT OUT: WHEN YOUR GIANT, RUDE BABY IS A PROCRASTINATOR

I'm due in two weeks, but I'm hoping she comes a little early!

—Everyone who has ever been pregnant

We all hope our babies come a little early, but they usually don't. Unfortunately, your due date is just an estimate; in fact, only 5 percent of babies are born on their due date, and most first babies are at least a few days (sometimes a couple of agonizing *weeks*) late. Your baby is very comfortable inside your body and will not develop empathy for several years after their birth, so they really give no fucks about how uncomfortable you are.

The end of pregnancy is pure hell, there's really no getting around it. You're stuffed to the gills with another human being, your entire body is filling with extra fluids in preparation for birth, and you can't leave the house without being chased through the Target parking lot by a mob of well-meaning strangers chanting "Any day now!" Each morning when you wake up and heave your enormous body into an upright position, your first thought is "Fuck, still pregnant." You're like a Judy Blume character, waiting for her period. Are you there, God? It's me, Giganto.

TO INDUCE, OR NOT TO INDUCE

Once you're full-term, you have the option to induce labor, and if the idea of waiting around for it to happen on its own sounds crazy-making, talk to your health-care provider about the benefits and risks of induction. We can't tell you whether you should induce labor, but we *can* tell you that you should never feel pressure to do so, unless there is an actual medical reason why you shouldn't wait. Should you induce? Short answer: if you want to.

If you've decided to wait this sucker out, here are a few tips to help you stay sane, even into week forty-two, when there's literally no room left for breathing and eating.

SOOTHING YOUR ANGRY BODY

Massage: Not only does massage feel good, but it's great for your body right now. Massage can help with fluid retention and swelling, stress relief, and emotional well-being. Maybe your partner is better than ours and they are willing to give you a massage that lasts more than seven minutes and uses both hands; good for you! If not, get thee to a professional trained in prenatal massage.

Walking: Unless you're some sort of CrossFit hero, walking is probably the most exercise you're doing at this point. It's good for you; it helps get your blood flowing, keeps your heart healthy, and at the end of pregnancy it is basically a strength-training exercise to haul that belly around your neighborhood. Too cold/hot/sunny/rainy/snowy/moody outside? Do like the old ladies do and strap those supportive sneakers on at the mall for a bit.

Live in your bathtub: If there was ever a time when it was legit okay to give up on life, it's now. Unless you have one of those bullshit tiny bathtubs from the 1950s, when human beings were apparently several feet shorter than they are now, your bath can be an oasis. Dump an entire bag of Epsom salts in there, and maybe some hippie oils. Light some candles, grab a very dumb novel or magazine, and tune the F out for a bit while you run out the clock.

Swimming: Weightlessness is delicious relief in late pregnancy; find a public pool, a private pool if you a fancy bytch, or hop your neighbor's fence in the middle of the night and float until you prune. Imagine you are a heartless procrastinator baby in a giant womb; you give no fucks. If you can find a place to do it naked, all the better.

Eating: Sometimes at the end of pregnancy, your health-care provider will get a little concerned about the size of your baby, and it's hard not to internalize this as you look back at forty-plus weeks of delicious cake-eating. Try to be kind to yourself; babies make you hungry. It's okay to eat food when you feel hungry. Trust your body and eat when you want to, with foods that make you feel good.

SOOTHING YOUR ANGRY MIND

Go on a date: It's sort of your last chance for a bit, so live it up and see a movie or hit up your favorite restaurant with your partner, or your best friend if you currently hate your partner for getting you into this mess in the first place. Often a relaxing activity will signal to your baby that it's time for them to come and ruin your relaxation.

Start a new book: The dumber the better; your brain is being sucked dry by your baby, so something easy to read and requiring very little brainpower is the perfect choice.

Binge-watch Netflix: Now is the perfect time to elevate those sausage legs, put on your granny glasses, and plow your way through every season of *Call the Midwife*. You'll laugh, you'll cry, you'll be glad you're not giving birth in Depression-era England. Just don't watch anything that's stressing you out—at all.

Have some lady time: Now is the time to hold court in your house and invite all your female friends to come take care of and distract you from the internal hell of your swelling body. Ask for pedicures and foot rubs in exchange for listening to their petty drama.

Take up a weird craft: The more useless, intricate, and antiquated, the better. Might we recommend quilling?*

Write: Someday you may look back on this time and smile, and if you write enough, you might find that you, like us, have enough notes to make a book proposal and write your own damn book. At the very least, getting the thoughts out of your head and onto paper is a release of pressure. And, girl, you got *pressure* right now. Write a letter to your baby, write a letter to yourself, write a list of things that hurt, write a list of things you're grateful for.

Complain: To your friends, to your partner, to strangers, to the internet, to literally anyone who will listen. If you are complaining to someone with a penis, you will most likely need to preface your complaints with the following: "I do not want your advice, and I do not want you to fix anything, because you can't. I just want to complain, and then I want you to massage me."

STILL PREGNANT?

Damn, girl. If you're looking to try to get this show on the road, check out "Natural Ways to Get Things Going" (page 101) for a myriad of methods to maybe induce labor, but probably not, sorry. Remember: no one in the history of womanhood has ever stayed pregnant forever.

---

* Rolling tiny pieces of paper into little coils and gluing them all together on a larger piece of paper to make an image. *Shrug.* It's a thing people do?

THE MANY VAGUE SIGNS OF LABOR

When the baby's coming, you'll know. In the weeks before that, you'll wonder, "Is this it?" as your body sends lots of vague signals that shit's about to go down. Here are some of the signs that *maybe* this is it.

STOMACH PAIN OR NAUSEA

Weird stomach pain or nausea could be related to early contractions. Or you could just be, you know, very pregnant.

BACK PAIN AND/OR CRAMPS

Contractions can definitely cause back pain. And if you're unfamiliar with the feeling of contractions, they can feel like a squeezing of your stomach, back, and entire torso. So if you're hurting, it might be a sign of the time, or just that your stomach has been weighing you down for several months now.

WANTING TO BE ALONE

Again, this could be another indication that you're very pregnant and cranky, but it could also mean you're ready to pop and want your privacy.

LOTS OF ENERGY

Some women report a burst of energy before labor, but it could just be that latte.

NO ENERGY

You might also feel exhausted right before labor. But people often do in late pregnancy, so who knows.

FLUSHED FACE

Malar flush is a rosy flush some women experience on their face right before they go into labor. But also, pregnant women can get very hot.

MORE CONCRETE SIGNS OF LABOR

Diarrhea or Vomiting

Many women will experience liquid poop, nausea, or vomiting at the start of labor. But it might also mean labor is a few days away. These signs aren't foolproof! If you can stomach it, try eating toast with jam or drinking something like soda to settle things. You don't want to go into labor dehydrated (though they can offer intravenous fluids at the hospital, if necessary).

Bloody Vaginal Discharge

The "bloody show" is when you expel a bloody bit of the mucus plug that has been sealing off your cervix. It is gross, but it's one of the surer signs that your body is making way for baby. Unfortunately it could still mean labor is days away.

Regular Contractions

If you're having strong contractions at regular intervals—this is probably it. Things could still stop and start for a while, but you're on your way. Real labor contractions (as opposed to Braxton-Hicks) occur within a somewhat predictable time period and start to get closer together over time.

Your Water Breaking or Leaking

Sometimes it's a gush of water and sometimes it's more of a slow trickle that will make you go, "Huh? Did I pee pee?" If you think your water's broken, call your obstetrician or midwife. Once it breaks there's a risk of infection, so if your membranes rupture prematurely (not accompanied by contractions) your health-care provider will want you to deliver within a day or two. This is not uncommon (10 to 15 percent of women experience their water breaking prior to contractions).

· · · · · · · ·

There you have it—all the unsure signs of labor. Good luck deciphering. Call your provider if you have concerns. And remember, when you know, you'll *really* know. No sense sweating it in advance (but we know you will).

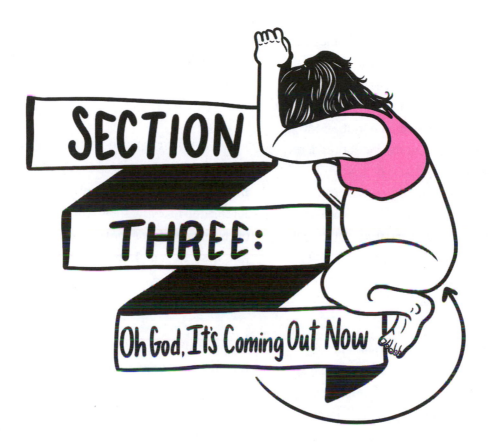

SECTION THREE: Oh God, It's Coming Out Now

THE START, STOP, WAIT

Even when you start going into labor, it's often unclear whether something's really happening. Early contractions feel different to different women, because some are more sensitive to the sensation, and the baby's position might affect where you feel the most pressure. The feeling is sort of a wave sensation, a gradual squeezing of the uterus that gains in intensity and then slowly dissipates. You might feel it in your abdomen (similar to a menstrual cramp) or your back or both places.

Since contractions often start slowly, or stop and start, it may take you a while to realize what's happening. You might find yourself saying, "I feel weird" for hours and hours until it finally clicks. You might think you're getting sick, or you're just really tired. Don't worry too much about figuring it out, because as we've said, once you know, you'll really know (so helpful, right?). As your contractions get stronger, you'll be able to feel them coming and can prepare yourself to get into the best physical position to handle the peak of the sensation.

> ## DID YOU FRIGGIN' KNOW?
>
> The uterine muscle is the largest muscle in a woman's body.[*] Ouch.

TIMING YOUR CONTRACTIONS

Once you've acknowledged that you're actually in labor, it's time to start timing your contractions so you know when to head to the hospital or have your doula and/or midwife head to you. There are two things to time: the duration of your contractions and the frequency.

Duration is the amount of time a contraction lasts from beginning to end. One thing to keep in mind if you were feeling unsure of your contractions early on is that you should start timing from the moment you feel tightening, even if it's not super painful or intense. If you discount the beginning of the wave of sensation, you may unintentionally underestimate the length and intensity of your contractions and become one of

---

[*] The largest muscle in a man's body is the nap muscle, which often spasms during early labor.

those people who gives birth in a car, like one of the authors of this book!*

Frequency is the amount of time from when one contraction begins and the next contraction begins. So your contractions are five minutes apart when one starts five minutes after the last contraction started. Do *not* start timing from the end of the contraction to the beginning of the next.

THE STAGES OF LABOR

The following are the stages of labor for vaginal delivery. You may not experience every stage if your labor is interrupted by an emergency cesarean, and you may not notice all the symptoms of each stage if you are on painkillers.

The **first stage** of labor is the bulk of your labor, from when your labor first starts until you are fully dilated to ten centimeters. It involves three stages.†

Early labor is the start of labor until when you are three centimeters dilated. This is when you should just try to chill and sleep if possible, though that's easier said than done. Contractions will be irregular, five to thirty minutes apart. This stage of labor can last for eight to twelve hours,‡ which is why it's often preferable to conserve energy and stay home for as long as your health-care provider deems safe.

Active labor is when you're dilated between four and seven centimeters. Contractions will get stronger, longer, and more regular, lasting forty-five to sixty seconds long and occurring three to five minutes apart. This is usually the time to head to the hospital. Active labor lasts for three to five hours on average.

Transition is when shit really starts hitting the fan. Thank the goddess, it is also the shortest stage of labor (thirty minutes to two hours). During this stage, your cervix will fully dilate. Contractions will last sixty to ninety seconds. You'll be wild-eyed and unconcerned about being buck-naked in a room

* Don't worry, this is pretty unlikely with a first birth, and giving birth in a car is not often as bad as it sounds (aside from the cleaning bill). If your labor is over before you get to the hospital, it means your labor is over. Yay!

† Wondering why they made the first stage of labor three stages instead of just making the whole thing five stages? SO ARE WE! We didn't make the rules.

‡ Keep in mind, these time frames are based on averages. Some labors progress very quickly. So make sure your support person is timing your contractions and keeping in touch with your health-care professional so that you know if you need to be in their care sooner rather than later.

full of strangers. This is when your support person must strike the delicate balance between fully supporting you and getting the fuck out of your way. If you're doing this unmedicated you may feel desperate and angry. This is the time to have one of those movie moments where you grab your partner by the collar or scrotum and make them fear for their life. Go for it!

THE RING OF FIRE / CROWNING

These are not references to medieval fantasy books but rather the moment when your baby's head starts to stretch out the opening of your vagina. You may feel a burning or stinging sensation, hence the "ring of fire." This is when you are likely to feel the urge to push, which feels a lot like having to poop. The amount of time varies, but with your first child it may take an hour or two for your baby's head to push its way out. Don't be scared by the aggressive terminology. In unmedicated labors, the pain of this pushing stage often pales in comparison to the pain of contractions preceding it. It's also a bit more exciting, so the pain may fade with the anticipation of meeting your baby.

The **second stage** of labor is when you literally deliver your baby. This often lasts between twenty minutes and two hours. You will feel a strong and at times unavoidable urge to push. You'll also feel pressure on your butthole as the baby presses into it.[*]

The **third stage** of labor is when you deliver the placenta. This is pretty easy compared to everything you've been through, aside from the fact that you're like, "I thought I was done already."

TRY TO KEEP A POSITIVE OUTLOOK EVEN THOUGH THIS IS HAPPENING

Contractions hurt—we're not gonna lie—but your mental outlook will greatly impact the way you perceive that pain. Think of each contraction as something getting you closer to meeting your baby, a hurdle you have to jump over. It also helps to try to think of your contractions as a very strong sensation, rather than a feeling of pain. A 2011 Oxford study[3] found that our perception of pain is influenced by expectation. For info on how to move through the pain, see "Trying to Stay Off the Drugs," page 101. For info on how to groove through the pain, see "When You Need All the Drugs," page 95.

* For more on pushing, see "The Weirdness of Labor" on page 130.

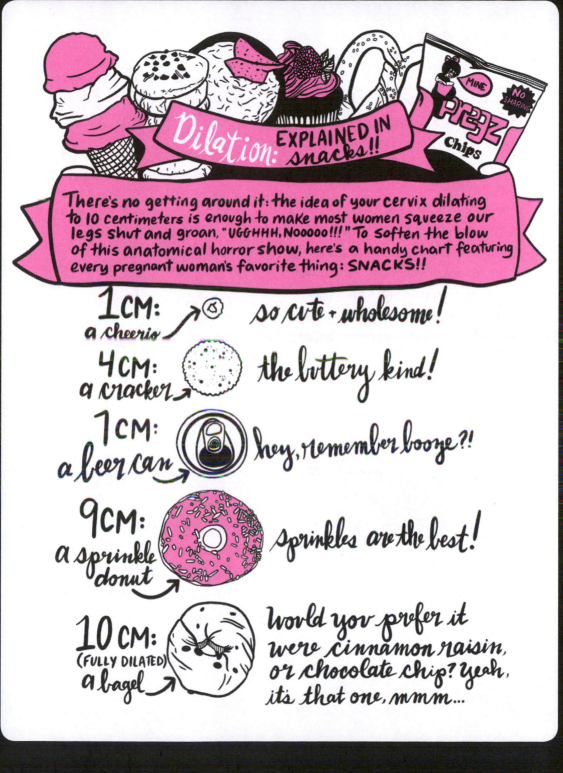

Dilation: EXPLAINED IN snacks!!

There's no getting around it: the idea of your cervix dilating to 10 centimeters is enough to make most women squeeze our legs shut and groan, "UGGHHH, NOoooo!!!" To soften the blow of this anatomical horror show, here's a handy chart featuring every pregnant woman's favorite thing: SNACKS!!

1CM: a cheerio — so cute + wholesome!

4CM: a cracker — the buttery kind!

7CM: a beer can — hey, remember booze?!

9CM: a sprinkle donut — sprinkles are the best!

10 CM: (FULLY DILATED) a bagel — Would you prefer it were cinnamon raisin, or chocolate chip? Yeah, it's that one, mmm...

THE WEIRDNESS OF LABOR

Birth is an otherworldly experience, beautiful *and* terrible. If pregnancy seemed weird, it's nothing compared to the sensory experience of having life spew from your loins. Many things you thought would be embarrassing during labor actually aren't, because holy shit, a person is coming out of you. If you're worried about having your vag flayed open for the world to see, worry no more. Here's some insane stuff you might experience during labor that you'll quickly shrug off amid all the chaos.

BACK LABOR

If the average labor is hell on earth, back labor is a trip to the actual bowels of hell. When the baby is not optimally positioned, it results in labor being more painful while taking longer to progress, since contractions are less efficient. Many women are still able to deliver vaginally even without meds, so don't panic if it's happening to you. You'll get through it one way or another. If that requires medical intervention, do what you gotta do. Back labor can sometimes be prevented by monitoring baby positioning.* But sometimes there are factors you can't control, like a baby that's dead set on destroying you.

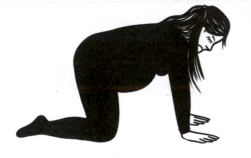

YOU MAY MOAN LIKE YOU'RE IN AN OVERACTED SEX SCENE

As we mentioned in "Trying to Stay Off the Drugs," an important part of labor is moaning through contractions like a wild woman. Moaning sounds insane, but it's one of the few things that really helps you get through the contractions. So go ahead and sound like you're having the loudest sex in the world with low, guttural moans.

* See "Getting Your Body Ready for Birth," page 76.

YOU MIGHT FALL IN LOVE WITH YOUR TOILET

Laboring on a toilet looked like nonsense in that hippie labor doc you watched. But when you're roaming around trying to find a comfortable laboring position, at some point you might want to just sit on the goddamn toilet and see how it feels. In later stages of labor, this lets you rest with your legs open, and use gravity to get that baby out. You can even make the toilet a little more comfy by putting towels on the seat edge or resting your head on a pillow on the back of the toilet as you straddle it. Don't worry, your baby's not gonna shoot into the toilet—someone will probably stop you if you're that far along.

YOU MAY BLEED, A LOT

You'll drip blood, either into a diaper or pad, or if you're stubborn and naked, all over the place the way God intended. Remember: you are a powerful goddess of creation, and everything that comes out of you is beautiful and should be framed, probably.

YOUR NORMAL BODILY URGES MIGHT BE QUIETED

During active labor, it can be a real challenge to stay hydrated or eat food to keep up energy, because our bodies concentrate so intensely on the task at hand (this is also why it's hard to pee!). Water during labor is cru-

cial, so anything that makes you thirsty is helpful. Have some sour candy or something salty around for your labor as long as your health-care provider deems it safe. Of course, the sight of any food at all may make you vomit. . . . So who knows, really?

YOU MIGHT WANT TO BE ALONE

There is a point in labor in which you will want to shut out the world, and that's when headphones will come in handy. "Goodbye, assholes!" you will growl, as you hit the play button on the hypnobirthing playlist / Sadé mix / Oprah podcast / Def Leppard discography. Girl, you know what you need.

DID YOU FRIGGIN' KNOW?

Popping babies out has a distinct aroma. You won't notice much while distracted by labor pains, but your partner probably will. It's not horrible, just specific. Like if you popped an enormous hot blister.

YOU MIGHT POOP

Pooping during labor is a thing that happens. The contraction of your uterus can cause a contraction of the intestines, and your urge to push might cause you to push out other stuff. This is a common fear of many women, but it's not a big deal. One of the people assisting your labor will wipe it up with swift nonchalance. You'll completely forget about it since you'll soon be distracted by the realization a whole person is coming out of your body. But your doula *will* know whether you've been eating all that flax seed she recommended.

YOU MAY HAVE VISIONS

It's not unheard of to have visions during labor. These might involve the sight of your future child, appearances from deceased relatives, or some animal/rainbow/voice-in-your-head that seems to be telling you that everything is going to be okay. If this sounds insane to you, move along. If it resonates with you, enjoy it. Anything that helps you feel calmer about this major life transition is a-okay in our book (this book). Your spiritual beliefs can be an incredible grounding force during pregnancy and childbirth.

YOU'LL GUSH LIQUID, MAYBE PEE

During labor, your water may break and make a big old mess. If your provider isn't there, make note of the time, color, and odor of the fluid. Greenish or brownish color (as opposed to clear) may indicate meconium (baby poop) in the fluid. This is often not an issue, but your provider will want to monitor to see if it's gotten into the baby's lungs. If it smells like pee, sorry—your baby probably just kicked you in the bladder.

YOU MAY REACH INSIDE YOURSELF TO TOUCH YOUR BABY'S HEAD

Sometimes providers will ask you to reach down and feel how close your baby is, in order to encourage you to keep going. It'll be weird and wet and smushy but also cool! Do it and realize you're *so* close.

YOU MAY SHAKE UNCONTROLLABLY

During or just after labor, it's very common for your body to start wildly shaking. "Why didn't someone tell me?" you'll think after wondering if you're having some kind of seizure. This is a normal reaction to hormonal shifts and adrenaline. You're fine. Your body is just like, "Whoa, I did it!"

Yes, You *Can* Wake Daddy

It's common to go into labor in the middle of the night or just before bedtime, at which point your health-care provider will probably tell you to try to get some sleep and rest up for the big event. At this point you will either (1) lie awake wondering if this is it, (2) fall asleep and wake up contraction-free the next day wondering what happened, or (3) lie awake having very painful contractions, wondering when you should wake up your annoyingly untroubled partner, as you internally and externally scream, "Hellooooo, I'm in labor over here!"

Some partners sleep blissfully through hour after hour of labor moans. It's a magical skill men especially seem to have. Many health-care providers will tell partners to rest up—labor can go on a long time and they get tired too, better to save their energy so they can help you through the main event—but we, the women who have actually in been in freakin' labor, say, "Fuuuck that bullshit." The choice of when to wake your partner depends on how soon you need to go to the hospital and how much their presence will help you in this difficult time. If things seem far along and/or you're too out of your mind in pain to time your own contractions, wake the motherfucker up. If the solitude is helping you achieve a sort of Zen connection to your labor, then let them be.

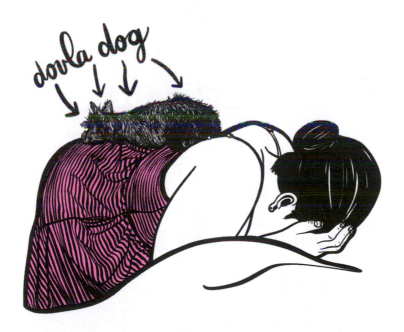

doula dog

Birthing Chairs: Horrible and Effective

The word "chair" is used loosely here, as there is a large hole where there would normally be a seat. Similar to laboring on a toilet without the association with poop, (although there may be poop involved, let's be honest), birthing chairs allow gravity to assist your labor and your muscles to work more efficiently.

Birthing chairs (or stools) have been around for thousands of years for a reason: though terrible for sitting, they work very well for birthing a baby. Their use can be traced all the way back to 1450 BC Egypt. Birthing chairs were a commonplace birthing tool until male physicians began dominating the field. Like most things worth loving, they began to experience popularity again in the 1980s, and many hospitals now provide them. Like most effective laboring techniques, laboring on one feels *terrible,* but it can significantly decrease the amount of time you spend in labor, and that's a good thing.

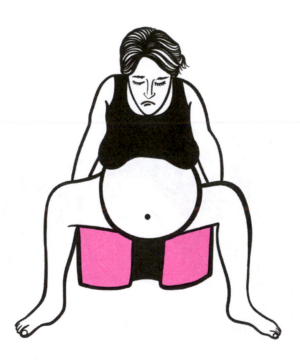

Documenting Your Birth

If a tree births another tree in the forest, but no one is there to artfully document it with high-res black-and-white photos that capture the emotion of the moment, did it even happen? In choosing how to document your birth, you have many options. Some families hire a professional photographer / videographer / birth stylist / social media guru, some give the sacred responsibility to their doula or partner, and still others don't think about this at all, and their midwives end up taking iPhone snaps with one hand while delivering their nearly ten-pound baby with the other.[*] Having a plan will take away some stress, so either delegate that shit, or pack your selfie stick. Do you.

Someone putting a camera in your face might be pretty off-putting during labor, but you might end up really loving this photo evidence of your triumph later. Of all the photos you'll look back on, the one of the moment you meet your baby is the money shot. Most moms say that this photo has the ability to transport them back to this happy moment like nothing else. Whether this happens in a birth pool at home, in the delivery room, or your baby gets whisked away to NICU and it takes a while, you'll have this moment, and it's worth documenting, gore and all.

. . . .

[*] A million thanks to my midwife, Nancy Giglio, for asking me to unlock my phone in the throes of labor so that I would have some pictures. —Jackie

Labor Positions

Moving around and trying different positions can help your baby move down the birth canal faster, which is good, because then labor will be over. Most labor positions don't have official names, so we've gone ahead and named them ourselves. No position works for everyone, so switch positions often and listen to your body. Remember, labor is like a shitty relationship: the more it hurts, the closer you are to the end! See the following pages for illustrated examples.

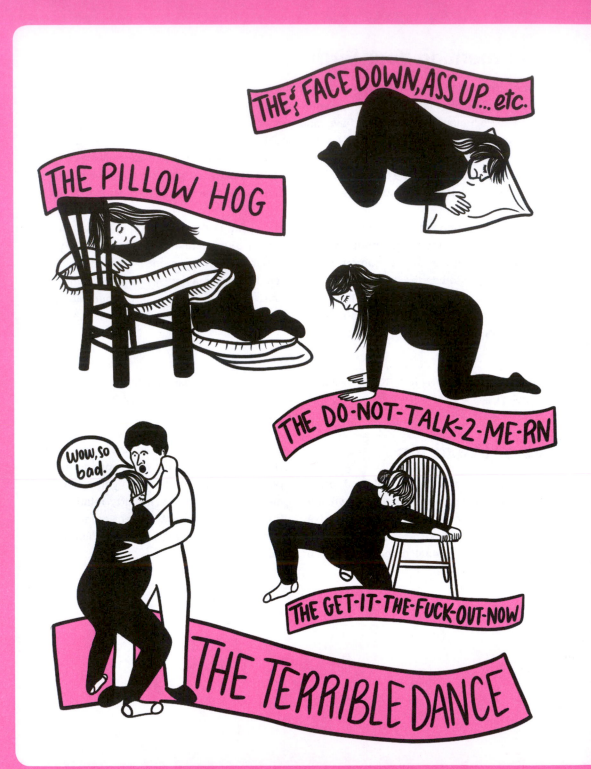

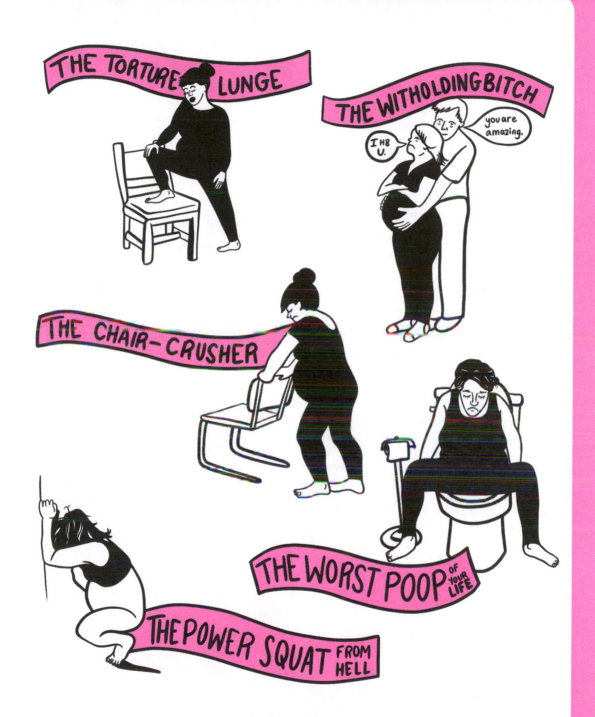

OKAY, SO NOW THE BABY IS OUTSIDE OF YOU

After the trauma and/or thrill of birth subsides and you've spent a few hours staring at the beautiful being before you, it hits you—holy shit, this is *really* happening. What do you do now that this thing is outside of you? What do you do when you realize . . .

THIS THING IS SO FUCKING TINY!

Babies are small, basically as small as humans get. You'll be pretty consumed by fears of harming one of the most delicate members of our species who are honestly so tiny it should be illegal for any of us to take care of them. You won't want to entrust your child to anyone, least of all yourself. In order to alleviate this state of constant fear, you have one thing to focus on:

* Sometimes referred to as "kangaroo care."

GET THAT BABY BIGGER

You'll do this with milk, either breast or formula. There are pros and cons to either (more on this later), but the key goal here is *keeping that baby alive.*

SKIN-TO-SKIN*

Assuming your baby doesn't require medical care, they'll probably be lightly wiped down and almost immediately placed on your chest. This is an efficient way of meeting your new favorite person, but it also offers health benefits. Direct contact with your skin comforts them, helps stabilize their body temperature, improves their ability to breastfeed and bond

SHE'S SO *CUTE?*

You're not the only one who's not feeling 100 percent right now; babies don't always come out as wide-eyed, plump little cherubs. Your alien-like baby might have a swollen face and a smushed head from the pressure of delivery and will be covered in a weird cheesy-looking substance called vernix. They may also look a bit skinny. For the first couple of months, your little monster may also develop baby acne, peeling skin, a lip blister from feeding, and gas so bad that they are clawing at their own face. Adorable!

If Your Baby Ends Up in the NICU

Ten to fifteen percent of babies born in the United States end up in a neonatal intensive care unit due to issues such as premature birth, birth defects, heart problems, infection, or breathing irregularities. Seeing your baby in an incubator or covered in tubes, IVs, and monitoring devices may be overwhelming, but we're lucky this technology exists and NICU center care is getting better all the time. If your pregnancy is very high-risk, it may be worth looking into surrounding hospitals to see what level of NICU care they provide. NICUs are rated numerically based on the availability of specialized equipment and which problems they can treat.

When a NICU baby is strong enough, you'll be able to hold them skin-to-skin outside the incubator. You may still be able to breastfeed or pump for your baby to be fed via a feeding tube or bottle. If you can't hold your baby, you can comfort them with your voice or by stroking them. Observe your baby to see what they respond to and what their different behaviors mean. Others are carefully watching out for baby, so remember to eat, drink water, and get rest. Once you're discharged from the hospital it's important to go home and recharge so that you're in a good place mentally to care for your baby going forward. Let yourself cry. Ask friends and loved ones for help with literally anything, including groceries, laundry, etc.

For comfort, you can tape a picture of yourself[*] to your baby's incubator or leave them with a small stuffed animal or item that has your smell on it. Make sure your cell phone numbers are prominently displayed near your baby's bed. Don't be afraid to ask the NICU nurses questions about your baby's care or whether you can hold or touch the baby. They are there for you too. Your pediatrician will likely visit your baby in the NICU and talk to the staff about the baby's needs, so trust that you're in good hands even after you leave the hospital.

* This also helps the NICU nurses recognize you when you come in.

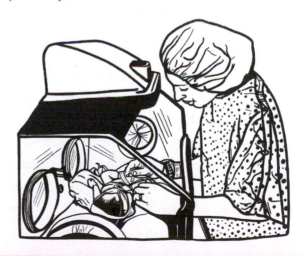

with you, stabilizes their breathing (perhaps because they hear your heart and breathing and start to mimic the rhythm), and can even help regulate their blood sugar.

You can continue skin-to-skin over the first couple of weeks as it also helps transfer good bacteria from your skin to your baby's. They don't have to be completely naked—a diaper is fine, and you can cover them with a blanket if the room is cold. Your baby will receive many of the same health benefits if your partner or someone else does this.

MORE DECISIONS YOU'RE GONNA HAVE TO MAKE UPON IMPACT

You'd think you were done after the baby is out, but there are a few more pressing calls you'll have to make regarding your baby. As silly as it sounds to keep repeating, we'll say it again—WE WON'T JUDGE YOU IF YOU DID THESE DIFFERENTLY. Well, mostly. We're like 99 percent not judging.

Cutting the Cord

Sometimes your provider will offer to let your partner cut the cord that attaches your baby to the placenta. This is one of those weird but kind of cool ways to get your partner in on the action of how miraculous and truly disgusting birth is. That cord is firmer and crunchier than it looks. Enjoy it if you're down!

Placenta Encapsulation / Placenta Magick

Okay, probably no one is forcing you to think about this, but you might be considering it. Placenta encapsulation is when someone (probably your doula or midwife) dehydrates your placenta, grinds it up, and puts it into capsules or a tincture for you to take later. This sounds insane, but some believe taking it can help you adapt to postpartum hormonal shifts, especially during breastfeeding and weaning, and help prevent postpartum depression. Currently, there is no research to back up these claims, and recent evidence suggests placenta pills can negatively affect milk supply. So go with your gut, and if your gut says, "I want to eat my own gut," you do you, witch lady! You'll need to tell your midwife or hospital staff so they can get the placenta into a cooler provided by you or your placenta-encapsulation person.

Eye Ointment

Ilotycin is an antibiotic ointment that is put in the eyes of newborns to prevent conjunctivitis (pink eye). It might seem weird to smear goop into a kid's eye practically the moment they're born, but there are common bacteria found in your genital and rectal area that can cause infection, which can progress rapidly and in some cases lead to blindness in newborns. You can delay applying for a few hours if you plan on nursing (the baby's vision may help him or her find your nipple in order to learn how to latch), and the goo will still get the job done.

To Bathe or Not to Bathe

You might assume you'd want to bathe your slimy baby after birth, and if you don't say anything, that's often what nurses will do at the hospital. But you actually don't have to. Many providers suggest postponing a baby's first bath, because the vernix covering their skin can help protect them from infection and absorb good bacteria from your body, while the stress of a bath can lower their blood sugar. If your baby isn't bathed, hospital workers must handle them with gloves to protect themselves from amniotic fluid and blood, which in turn protects your baby from any viruses they might be harboring. If your labor was especially messy,[*] you may want to go for the bath, but know you often have the option to refuse. After that, you should really only sponge bathe your baby in the first few days, since the umbilical cord is still drying up.

. . . .
[*] We're talking poop.

Finding a Pediatrician

Seemingly as soon as you head home from the hospital,[*] you must take your baby to the pediatrician, who will check them out, weigh them, and marvel at that one weird birthmark/cowlick/webbed toe.

You'll want a doctor with the right balance of invested and chill, who'll inform rather than shame you, and who's also a good fit for your level of interest in alternative medicine and nontraditional lifestyles. Are you vegetarian? Planning international travel as a family? Having a nonalarmist doctor who's aware of the specific needs of your family is ideal.

Location is a major factor for doctors, because you don't want to be shuttling your kid an hour away when they get sick. You want someone who won't let you do anything dangerous but also will trust you and give you a doctor's note to take them back to daycare when you're on a work deadline and they seem totally fine. Decent hours and a responsive staff are essential when you're trying to get forms filled out for daycare and school. So ask around, read online reviews, and take your best shot. You can always change doctors later.

. . . .
[*] Generally, when your baby is three to five days old.

Vaccines

Most vaccines are not given until your baby's two-month checkup, though they will probably offer the first dose of the hepatitis B vaccine at the hospital. If you don't want to do it then, you can do it at their first pediatrician visit. While it's painful to see your baby get a needle, it's nothing compared to exposing your child and other children to curable and sometimes deadly diseases.

Since there's a lot of misinformation out there about vaccines causing autism, here are the facts as we know them: at this time, there are thousands of documented preventable deaths from failure to vaccinate, and zero autism diagnoses scientifically linked to receiving a vaccine. Some children do suffer from immune diseases and other conditions that prevent them from receiving vaccines, which is why it is important for healthy children to receive vaccines in order to create "herd immunity"—when most of the population is immunized, contagious diseases cannot spread to those who aren't.

Despite all of this, it's hard to argue that the pharmaceutical industry is trustworthy; we deserve more accountability and transparency from an industry literally drowning in money, especially one with such an important role in the health of all Americans. Until we get that, do your research. There are ways to be medically conservative while still vaccinating your child, such as resisting the urge to "get the next vaccine over with" when you go into the pediatrician for a sick visit; the effects of vaccinating a child while their immune system is lowered are still not well known.

If your partner has a stronger stomach, send them in with the baby for shots while you wait outside. Don't worry, you're still a good mom! Also, if you're breastfeeding, feeding your baby immediately after the vaccine or while they're getting it will comfort them, and possibly even reduce pain, due to the release of oxytocin. It'll be over before you know it.

Vitamin K Shot

Vitamin K shots are mandatory in some states and are generally given in other states unless the parent asks for an exception. These shots prevent brain bleeds caused by vitamin K deficiency. Like vaccines, this momentary and minor pain for your baby is worth fending off a rare but horrible outcome. Science is good.

Circumcision

Yep, deciding whether to cut off part of your son's penis is a thing. Weird, right? If you have cultural reasons for doing it, cool—that's your right. Circumcision has certain health benefits related to infection and STDs, *but a* similar level of prevention can be obtained through basic hygiene and use of a condom, so if you don't want to cut the genitals of your newborn baby, don't worry—you're not some anti-science nut. Also, from what we've heard, having a foreskin makes sex more pleasurable for both male and female partners. Some argue a boy's junk should look like his father's, but since many of us look unlike our parents, it might be better to teach kids self-acceptance rather than conformity. All that said, please do not go to town attacking people who did circumcise. It's not the same as female circumcision.

Naming Your Baby!

You've probably prepared for this, but sometimes the shock of the birth makes you re-think everything, particularly if "she just doesn't look like a Cassandra." You're allowed to throw everything out the window and make impulsive decisions, even if you've already hung adorably crooked hand-painted wooden letters over Cassandra's crib. Your kid will be stuck with this name for the rest of their life, listen to your gut.

· · · · · · · ·

These are a lot of decisions to make when you're also recovering from childbirth, so you may want to research in advance and make a list of choices for your support person to have on hand. Talk to your ob-gyn or midwife to make sure you're on the same page and know their policies.

Recovering from a Vaginal Birth (Don't Look Down)

After vaginal birth, your vagina et al is best left alone. The postmortem can wait. But if you're like us, let's be honest, you're probably gonna look. Things will be . . . stretched, sore, and swollen.

TEARING

Vaginal tears are not a given, but they're not uncommon, especially for first-time moms. Don't worry, they sound more serious than they are and often heal pretty quickly. There are a couple of different types:

Labial Tears

Labial tears occur on the labia (the flesh flaps on the side of your vagina) and sting like crazy when you pee. They can range from surface abrasions to deeper lacerations. Because of location they cannot be stitched up, and there's not much to do besides wait for them to heal and squeeze water on them when you pee (more on this later).

Perineal Tears

Perineal tears occur on the perineum (the area between your vagina and butthole). Minor perineal tears (first-degree or superficial) are generally not as painful as labial tears because the wound can be sewn shut by your doctor or midwife and is not getting moved around as much or flushed by your fiery pee. Second-degree perineal tears are when the muscle is also torn. These take longer to sew up and heal and can be more uncomfortable. Third- or fourth-degree tears extend into the muscle of your anus, and discomfort may last for three or more months, but these are fairly unlikely.

While tears are annoying, they can be healed. If pain persists, contact a pelvic-floor physical therapist, an expert on postpartum PT for your vag, who can help you learn how to break up scar tissue and get that puss back in good workin' order.

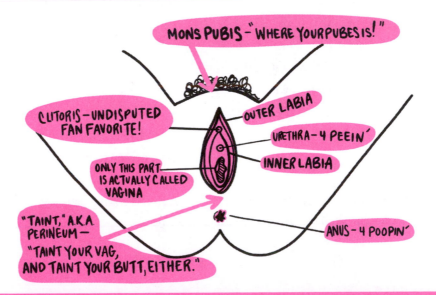

MONS PUBIS – "WHERE YOUR PUBES IS!"

CLITORIS – UNDISPUTED FAN FAVORITE!

ONLY THIS PART IS ACTUALLY CALLED VAGINA

OUTER LABIA

URETHRA – 4 PEEIN'

INNER LABIA

"TAINT," A.K.A. PERINEUM — "TAINT YOUR VAG, AND TAINT YOUR BUTT, EITHER."

ANUS – 4 POOPIN'

HAPPY BIRTHDAY, BODY DESTROYER!

The ongoing theme of motherhood is "Oh, you thought that was bad, wait'll you see what's in store!" Just when you thought you'd had all the terrible pregnancy symptoms, your little one makes a last-ditch attempt to really wreck your body. Luckily, most of the physical trauma of labor is recoverable. Here's what you might be in for.

YOUR NONRESTORATIVE CONVALESCENCE

Unless you birthed deep in the woods, you'll probably have a lot of interruptions early on. At the hospital, nurses will do check-ins, regularly interrupting your sleep. Sometimes they'll do this gently and quietly. Sometimes they need the lights on to take your vitals or are just being assholes about it. It's tiring. And if you also have visitors, it can drive you to tears. If you're losing your shit, ask everyone to leave you alone so you can get some rest.

Butt 'Roids

Like tears, the idea of hemorrhoids coming out of your butt is terrifying before having a baby. *Butt* once you've experienced them, they're often not that big a deal. Hemorrhoids are stretched and swollen veins in the anus and lower rectum, often occurring after trying to push a baby out, or you might already have them simply from being pregnant and constipated. Sometimes you can feel them near your butthole, or they might be inside where you can't. Symptoms range from unnoticeable to itching to painful. You might notice small amounts of blood when you poop. The ice diapers we mention later in this chapter can help, as can smaller witch-hazel pads used to wipe after you go to the bathroom. These are often provided at the hospital and can be found at the drugstore. You can also place baking soda on the area to alleviate itching. Get plenty of water and fiber to avoid straining while you poop.

Cramping

After birth, your uterus has to contract down from its enormous size to its original size. It'll do this pretty quickly in order to expel the placenta and other fluids, which can leave you feeling a bit crampy. Your health-care team will try to help this along in order to prevent large blood clots from forming.

Sometimes they'll give you Pitocin, but almost always they'll give you the worst massage ever, kneading your stomach very hard right after birth and sometimes a couple of times after that.

Lochia

Expect several weeks of bloody vaginal discharge, which goes by the fittingly disgusting term "lochia." This will happen even if you had a C-section. It's incredibly annoying to be changing menstrual pads, breast pads, diapers, and everything else you and your baby are currently leaking on, but it's a good reminder that you're still healing. The place where your placenta detached from inside your uterus is basically an open wound. So slow down as much as you can for a few weeks while you take care of yourself and your baby. Lochia will be dark red in the first few days, pinkish for a few more after that, and then whitish yellow. If you try to do too much, you may find the brighter blood reappears or does not decrease over time. Keep an eye on it and talk to your provider if you have concerns.

Floppy Belly

After the baby is out of you, your belly deflates into a loose sack of flesh. It'll seem suddenly so much smaller and yet . . . not. Try to laugh about how ridiculous it is in addition to all the weird things going on with your body. It'll slowly firm up over time, and right now you need to rest as much as humanly possible. Try not to judge your postpartum body—that floppy sack of flesh grew an entire human.

C-SECTION RECOVERY*

C-sections are major abdominal surgery, and there are some things about C-section recovery that will look different from a vaginal birth (besides your vagina, which will look different in a good way!).

Recovering in the Hospital

After your baby is born, your legs are going to be numb for longer than you expect, and this is a normal side effect of the anesthesia. Since you'll be pretty loopy, you might need to be reminded that they are still there, so designate one person in your post-op room as the "leg reminder."

"No, you have legs. They're right here," they will say, and stab a finger into your numb, stubbly calves.

"*Oh*, phew," you still say, and pass back out for a little while. Repeat as necessary.

At some point nurses will come in and

....
* For info on what to expect when you have a C-section, see page 152.

Becoming a Vagina/Butt/Boob Witch

There is so much going on with your body that you'll feel like a witch mixing potions to heal her ravaged form. Here are some magical tools to have on hand.

ICE DIAPERS! (WITCH-HAZEL PADS)

You know those giant overnight maxi pads with wings that you haven't worn since the summer you got your period at camp and it was all they had at the infirmary? Buy those; the bigger the better. Douse them in witch hazel (the rose-scented one is delightful) and freeze each one separately (or they will stick together) in a plastic bag. Your bruised and angry future vagina thanks you in advance. Witch-hazel pads soothe your vagina and ease swelling. However, witch hazel can sting labial tears. If that's the case, stick to plain ice packs.

PERINEAL IRRIGATION BOTTLE

This magical tool is basically a glorified ketchup squeeze bottle, like you'd find at a roadside barbecue stand, but it's sterile and clear and you fill it with water. Aim the water directly at your sore parts, start spraying before the stream of pee begins, and you'll avoid the stingy postpartum pees. The hospital will provide this, or you can order online for home birth.

NIPPLE SALVES

There are a variety of products designed to cool and protect your nipples as your baby is learning to latch and inadvertently chewing the shit out of them. If you plan to breast-feed, have some on hand since your tired partner will get the wrong thing when you send them to five stores in search of "some kind of nipple junk."

Hot tip: postpartum showers can go from feeling *so* good to *so so* bad when your nipples are raw, since hot water can irritate them further. Slather your nipples in a petroleum or lanolin-based ointment (because it's water-resistant) before your shower and you'll protect your tender-AF nips from further upset. Apply some more when you get out. Don't worry—nipple ointment is safe for babies to ingest. Try to keep other lotions and products away from your nipples, since they may not be safe for your baby.

ABDOMINAL BINDER

That sack of a belly isn't the only thing hanging loosely from your frame; pretty much everything in your abdomen feels weirdly loose. Your body is still pumped full of relaxin, making your pelvic area feel unstable, and your recently squished-into-a-corner organs are now all "WTF, there's so much space in here!" Abdominal-binder belts are often marketed to help you "lose the baby pooch" or some other offensive variation of body shaming, but false advertising aside, stabilizing your pelvis and swaddling your organs tight can really help your body "come back together," and that feels good.

IBUPROFEN

Your nurse or midwife will probably offer you ibuprofen right after labor. Take all of it as often as prescribed. You might still be in a state of shock, or full of other medications, but once that wears off, you'll wish you'd taken the ibuprofen. Your body is bruised, to say the least, and headaches might be a side effect of other meds you've been on.

STOOL SOFTENERS

If you're offered stool softeners by your provider, you should probably take those too, especially if you undergo a C-section, have perineal stitches, or hemorrhoids. You may feel constipated for various reasons, including drugs and hormones, and they often won't let you leave the hospital unless you've farted or pooped. Yup, get used to being asked about that.

What to Forage from the Hospital

As you leave the hospital, steal everything that isn't bolted down! Diapers, wipes, diapers, pads, creams, mesh undies, and all the diapers. The hospital will throw out most of this if you don't use it. And they pretty much expect you to snag whatever you can lay your hands on. Above all, make sure to grab that perineal irrigation bottle (small plastic bottle used to shoot water at your vagina while you pee). If you have any tears, it will sting like hot flames when you pee, and the water counteracts the acidity of your urine. You may be somewhat numb at first, so bring that magical little twenty-five-cent bottle home. Your partner will have a hell of a time finding one at the store when you realize you want it later.

change all the pads covering your incision and your vagina and clean you up a bit. Unfortunately, with C-sections you'll still have the lochia of a vaginal delivery, so you'll have to wear pads to absorb that too. Nurses will bring weird disposable mesh hospital underwear to hold everything in place. There may be a disturbing amount of blood pouring out of you the first time you stand up after surgery, because gravity. This is normal.

You may not be able to move for a day or two after surgery, and luckily you won't have to, thanks to a catheter channeling away all your pee, but it's a good idea to get up as soon as you can in order to get the blood flowing and help prevent blood clots. The first time you stand up, it will burn like fire, and this is normal and apparently even a *good sign* of nerve health. It will be hard to walk, because obviously. Once you're able to stand for longer stretches, you'll be able to take a shower, which may help you feel better overall. Don't worry—the water should not hurt your incision. If you have staples you should wait about a week before taking a bath. And don't scrub around your incision.

It's common for one side of your scar to be more painful than the other, and to feel like your organs have been pulled out and then put back in a slightly different place, because they *were*. You'll get used to it, we promise. An abdominal binder can really help minimize this creepy feeling and help stabilize your wobbly body so you're in less pain. They'll probably give you some type of wrap in the hospital, and you can continue to wear it for a while after.

Keep taking the meds they give you and let hospital staff know if you're not feeling good, because they may be able to try different meds. The discomfort of C-section recovery varies from woman to woman, with many claiming it is really not that bad. If you're not feeling great, there is often something that can be done about it.*

Before you leave the hospital, channel your inner bandit/hoarder and steal as many pairs of adult diaper underwear as you can stuff in your hospital luggage. You'll want to avoid elastic-waisted undies for a while, because the elastic will sit right on your scar.

Due to lochia, going commando is not really an option, so you can either buy enormous loose granny panties or special C-section undies that compress your incision in order to reduce swelling. These often have an adjustable fit.

In addition to the physical trauma of birth, you'll feel the emotional impact of the physical stress you've been under. Any way you feel about your birth is valid. You're allowed to be sad. You're allowed to be proud of your birth. You're allowed to feel a mix of everything. Remember, pregnancy primes your body to heal faster than usual, so you will recover from most of the damage fairly quickly. Despite the heady mix of pain and hormones, much of this will be over before you know it. And you can get help for issues that linger.

* Some women are hesitant to complain about pain after not delivering vaginally, because they feel as if they didn't "do birth correctly." No, girl. C-sections are major abdominal surgery. You're a warrior—get you some pain drugs.

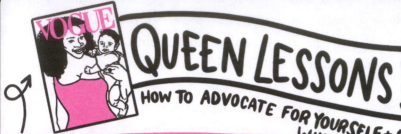

QUEEN LESSONS w/* SERENA

HOW TO ADVOCATE FOR YOURSELF + OTHER WOMEN WHEN NO ONE IS LISTENING.

In 2018, Vogue published an interview with tennis star/ mom goddess Serena Williams, describing her experience with an all-too-common issue in women's health: the alarming propensity among health-care providers to doubt the experiences of women and our knowledge of our own bodies.

A LIL' BACKSTORY: IN 2011, SERENA UNDERWENT SURGERY FOR TREATMENT OF A BLOOD CLOT IN HER LUNGS, ALSO KNOWN AS A PULMONARY EMBOLISM (P.E.). THE CLOT FORMED AS A RESULT OF A PRIOR SURGERY ON HER FOOT.

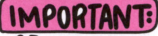

IMPORTANT: P.E. IS <u>VERY</u> RARE. YOU ARE FINE + HEALTHY. CHILL.

BUT ANYWAY...

In 2017, after an emergency C-section during the birth of her daughter, she felt the familiar symptoms of P.E. and urgently requested a CT scan and a blood thinner. The nurses on call told her that her pain meds were making her "Confused." It took several tries with different hospital staff before anyone would listen, and when they finally agreed to run the CT scan they found—you guessed it—blood clots in her lungs again. She finally got the blood thinner she had initially asked for, and ~~it saved her life~~ she saved her own life.

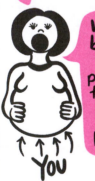

You

WOW, are you bitches trying to scare a pregnant woman to DEATH?! Why are you telling me this RIGHT NOW?

To empower you. While P.E. is rare, Complications during labor + postpartum are not. Because it's so common for women to feel unheard at the doctor, it's also common to feel helpless when you know something is not right with your body, and no one is listening to you. This is when you will need to summon your INNER SERENA and advocate for the care you deserve. No woman should have to fight so hard to be heard, but here we all are. At least we are together? Speaking of which...

WE ARE ALL IN THIS TOGETHER

#MOMS

All women deserve better care, but some women among us are treated better than others, and this needs to change. We are all mothers; this unites us. Together we are legion, and we can change this shit.

FIRST...

A QUICK HEADS-UP

If you're a white lady like us, and this is new info for you, you'll probably have some big feelings while reading this. Feel them, girl; they will transform you into a powerful good witch. We have work to do, and it's becoming pretty clear that women are gonna be the ones to do it.

If you're a woman of color:
1. We are with you.
2. We see you.
3. We are so very sorry.

Shitty Truths

BACKED BY ENOUGH DATA TO CHOKE YR RACIST UNCLE!

☑ Women of color (especially black women) are statistically much more likely to have their experiences + self-knowledge doubted.

☑ Black + Latinx patients are 22% LESS LIKELY TO BE GIVEN PAIN MEDS than white patients presenting with the same complaints. WTF.

☑ A recent study found that black women in NYC were 12x MORE LIKELY TO DIE IN CHILDBIRTH than white women, and this alarming statistical gap is WIDENING, not shrinking.

If a millionaire tennis star was not believed when she tried to advocate for herself, where exactly does that leave women w/ less resources?

WHEN TO ADVOCATE ♥

FOR YOURSELF OR SOMEONE ELSE!

☑ DURING PREGNANCY, LABOR, OR POSTPARTUM WHEN YOU DON'T FEEL HEARD.

☑ WHEN YOU SEE THIS HAPPEN TO SOMEONE ELSE.

☑ WHEN YOUR DOC SAYS SOMETHING IS NORMAL BUT IT DOESN'T FEEL NORMAL, AND NONE OF YOUR MOM FRIENDS HAVE THE SAME ISSUE.

☑ WHEN YOUR DOC SUGGESTS SOMETHING THAT MAKES YOU UNCOMFY.

☑ WHEN YOU ARE IN "ANY" WAY UNHAPPY WITH THE CARE YOU ARE RECEIVING. YOU. ARE. NOT. ANNOYING. FOR. NEEDING. HELP.

HOW2 ADVOCATE:

1. DO. NOT. SHUT. UP. Until someone listens. Ask for supervisors, call hospital administrators. Enlist your support network to help you; more voices = louder.

2. Take notes + keep records. If a doctor brushes off your concerns, say:

THIS DUDE WILL RUN TESTS.

"I'd like a note in my chart that says I came in with these issues and you've decided not to run tests. I'll wait."

3. Know your rights. If you're doing a hospital birth, know their policies and know what you can decline + request. HOLD THEM TO THIS.

4. Share your experiences with other moms, but also with men + other health-care professionals, and really anyone who will listen. We can change this.

5. Vote with your vag. Elect officials who support better health care and are pro-choice.

After a C-Section

Listen, superhero, stay in bed for as long as they tell you to stay in bed, longer if necessary. Most doctors will tell you to do this for about a week, with a little bit of getting up and walking around daily. A combination of bed rest and short periods of movement will keep your blood flowing. Without a motorized hospital bed, sitting up and getting out of bed will be hard for a while, so ask for help, and never push through sharp pain. Propping yourself up with a ton of pillows helps, especially if you're attempting to breastfeed in bed.

You should not be lifting anything heavier than your baby, pushing, pulling, or doing deep bends for six to eight weeks, or until your incision is completely healed. Most women are instructed not to drive for several weeks. If you'd like to extend this period of rest beyond the six- to eight-week mark and milk it for all it's worth (which we enthusiastically support), just cross this paragraph out with Sharpie so your partner doesn't read it, and tell him it said something mean about husbands that you didn't agree with. But if it makes you feel better, you should be fully recovered from your C-section in about six weeks. You've got this! Here is some other information and advice:

STAY HYDRATED

This is important for all new moms, but especially those taking narcotic pain medication while healing from a C-section. Pain medication is infamous for causing consti-

pation, and straining to poop is *definitely* not something you need to add to your to-do list right now. Guzzle as much water as you can stand, and think about eating foods rich in fiber and magnesium to keep those artfully rearranged bowels a-flowin'. Take stool softeners or a suppository if you're offered them. Your OB may even prescribe laxatives to take home. You may have very intense gas pains as your bowels start working again.

BE PATIENT WITH BREASTFEEDING

You can begin trying to breastfeed pretty much as soon as you meet your baby, but it may be a challenge. Have someone help you lift the baby, and try using a support pillow so you don't have to put as much pressure on your abdomen. You may also want to try a football hold, where the baby is tucked under your arm and off to the side, or a side-lying position. Breastfeeding is a challenge for most new moms, but especially those recovering from surgery. It may take a little longer for your milk to come in, so don't hesitate to supplement with formula so that you don't have to worry about your baby's bilirubin* levels. A bit of formula in the first few days does not mean you're going to have to use formula forever.

DEALING WITH SORENESS

In addition to everything else, you're also healing from having a catheter in your urethra. So awesome, right? Slather a bunch of ointment with pain reliever in it onto your

---

* For more on bilirubin, see page 171.

urethra to help the pain. Keep the area clean, and drink water like it's your other new job* to prevent a UTI, though it basically already feels like you have one.

YOUR SCARS WILL HEAL

It's normal for your scar to be itchy/numb for several weeks, because incisions sever nerves and it takes time for them to regrow. You may also have a weird "shelf" of skin and fat above the scar, which will eventually chill out and look less weird, but it takes time.

Around six weeks, your scar should be completely healed, barring complications. Once it is, it's a good idea to massage it with oil. This will *not* feel good, but it will help increase blood flow to the area, which will aid in healing the parts you can't see, and eventually make the scar less visible. You can also get silicone scar sheets at the drugstore. Honestly though, scars are a badass reminder of the fact that your perfect baby came out of your perfect body perfectly; you are perfect.

* * * * * * * * * *
* You are also a mom now, remember? Damn those are some good pain meds!

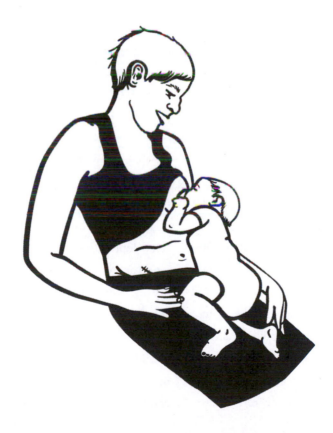

YOUR BIRTH RECOVERY PLAN

Listen, babies are very distracting. They're very small and smell very good, and they need almost constant attention from at least two people. They make you deliriously happy and deliriously tired, so to stay happy and healthy you need a solid self-care plan in place before you give birth.

Since the crazy chemicals and love hormones that your body produces will make it very hard for you to concentrate on yourself, you'll need help sticking to this plan. Take a picture of your plan and text it to your partner and make them go to the copy shop and print several copies. Hang a copy on the fridge so that when the people ask you how they can help you during postpartum you can just point at it with your elbow and grunt as you wash an endless stream of bottles and pacifiers. Early motherhood is a beautiful slog, and the postpartum period is a period of recovery, especially if you've had surgery.

"I got this," you'll probably say, as you pour baby formula into your coffee and wipe up some errant vomit with a balled-up nursing bra that you found in the refrigerator.

Trust: you don't got this, and you're not supposed to. It's impossible to do it all, so let other people help you *whenever* they offer, and if they don't, ask them. Here are some things you will need to make space for postpartum.

SLEEP, TRUST US, *SLEEP*

People love to tell you how important it is to "sleep when the baby sleeps," like it's some ancient, easy-to-follow wisdom. The truth is, this became a colloquialism *waaaaay* before we began to acknowledge the powerful and natural anxiety that comes along with motherhood, which makes it very hard to follow these instructions.

It's hard to sleep when your baby sleeps, for a number of reasons. Hormones make you crazy like a protective animal, plus you need to do lots of other stuff that you can't do while holding a newborn, like shower and poop and pluck your damn eyebrows and stare at your perfect baby, etc., etc.

Here's the thing though: long periods of sleep deprivation have devastating effects on mood and can cause anger, irritability, memory loss, confusion, depression, and relationship issues. Having a new baby is not anything like college finals week, or that time you had a wild weeknight and never slept and just drank a giant Red Bull and went to work; you cannot power through several *years* of poor sleep. Yes, it may be years before your child learns to fully embrace sleep, but that doesn't mean you need to go without. It just means you need help.

Let people hold your baby when they come over. Trust us, you're not missing anything. While they hold the baby, resist the urge to find some sort of housework to complete or to serve your guests in any way. Instead, say these simple words: "I need to nap. Thank you, goodbye." This also works on your partner. In the beginning, it is tempting to want to band together and do everything "as a family," but this often means that no one sleeps and usually means lots of "yelling as a family." Take turns resting—the time you spend as a family will be much higher in quality.

How to Nap

Go to your bedroom. Turn off all lights and devices and televisions. Stay. Off. Your. Phone. Draw the shades and do whatever else you can to create an environment conducive to napping. Stay. Off. Your. Phone. Sniff some lavender, wear a sleep mask, use a sound machine, masturbate, do whatever you need to do in order to make a nap happen, and don't come back until you feel a little bit more rested. Seriously, stay off your phone; even if you can't sleep, resting your eyes for thirty minutes is a much better alternative to staring at a screen and consuming information like a robot powered by anxiety. Don't feel guilty if you didn't sleep. You rested, right? You weren't looking at your phone?

NOW IS THE TIME FOR SELF-CARE

When we compare ourselves to the rest of the world, it's embarrassingly clear: America sucks at caring for postpartum mothers. All over the world, the traditions vary, but the methodology is the same: to honor and support a woman's transition into motherhood and allow her the time, space, tools, and community necessary to experience a full recovery from birth and ensure a successful and happy future. While the rules vary across communities, women are most often sent to bed while the other women in the community care for her, run the home, and allow her time to bond with her baby and rest.

Latin America calls it *cuarantena*, China has *zuo yuezi*, Japan calls it *ansei*, which means "peace and quiet and pampering." In Korea it lasts one hundred days, in India it's sixty days, and in Jamaica it's eight days. Most cultures incorporate self-care rituals like herbal baths, massage, and uterine-binding to help organs return to their original positions inside the body. America is like, "Nah, you're fine. Want some Zoloft, crazy pants?"

Don't let American culture gaslight you though, booboo. You are a goddess and deserve to be treated as such. Get in your bed and bark orders to whoever will listen; fuck the patriarchy, welcome to the matriarchy. It starts whenever you want it to. Rest your body, hang with your baby, let someone else worry about the rest of it.

PAMPER YOURSELF

Postpartum bodies feel really weird, and for good reason. During pregnancy, your body is full of extra blood and hormones and fluid and life-supporting chemicals. After birth, not only do you lose all that extra blood and fluid pretty quickly, but over the first year your body experiences several hormonal free falls,[*] as levels attempt to return to (a new) normal. If you're breastfeeding, you're also being *literally drained* of your life source day and night, and usually on very little sleep.

Anything you can do to make your weird body feel more like itself is good, so take a minute to consider which grooming habits feel like an important part of your ritual. It's hard to remember these things when you're tired, so write them down and refer back when you're like, "Wow, my body feels like hot garbage baking in the sun, WTF should I do?"

YOU DESERVE TO HEAL

Birth injuries are pretty much standard, and many of them fall by the wayside after the birth is over, never getting fully resolved. This is not cool *or* necessary; you deserve to heal fully, and unfortunately you will probably need to advocate for yourself to make that happen. A birth injury can take many forms; some of us tear during birth, some of us need pelvic-floor strengthening work to stop leaking pee when we cough, and some of us need mental health treatment to deal with the trauma of all the changes that have ravaged us. All of these birth injuries are normal and valid and can heal.

Be a squeaky wheel; if something hurts, complain. Pregnancy and birth may be natural, but it's still an intense time of injury and recovery, and it wreaks absolute havoc on our bodies and our minds. In *less than one year* our uterus takes over most of the space inside our abdomen and squishes all our other organs, weird hormones make us bend and stretch and loosen in ways that completely change our posture and center of gravity and alignment, we gain weight *very fast*, our hormones make our brains *weird*, and then toward the end someone starts punching and kicking us harder and harder from the *inside* until they force their way out

* RIP, Tom Petty.

of our body through a tiny exit, or are cut out of our abdominal wall in a major surgery. After it's over, you will likely have some issues that need addressing, both physically and emotionally. If you feel self-conscious or dramatic about this, try to remind yourself of all of the man colds* you have witnessed in your life.

Whatever your birth injury, there is treatment available. In France, postpartum pelvic physical therapy is a standard part of women's health care, and it should be standard here too. Many ob-gyns and midwives do not inform women of the efficacy of such treatment because they are not well versed in it, but if you're in pain, go to PT. Try chiropractic, acupuncture, massage, or myofascial release. Postpartum is a great time to experiment with new self-care habits and see which ones make you feel better. If something isn't working for you, drop it and try something new, but *keep at it* until you are healed.

GET MOVING

Starting slow is key, but once you're cleared by a medical professional to resume (ha!) exercising, start stretching and moving your body and you'll start to feel better. For a short while it will be easy to exercise around your sleepy immobile baby, but eventually your baby won't want you to do anything without holding them, so set up an exercise routine so that the space you need to take care of your healing body does not evaporate. Many gyms have free or affordable daycare, where a slightly hungover college student will hold your baby while you do cardio, and this is a *blessing*.

If you've never had an exercise routine before, you are certainly not alone. Postpartum is a great time to start new habits, since babies explode your entire life structure, making it easy to start from scratch. Tune in to your body and listen to what it needs. Feel tight? Stretch it out with some postpartum yoga. Feel weak? Strength training will help. Spending hours on the couch bent over and breastfeeding? Go for a long walk and concentrate on standing tall and engaging your core, which probably feels like it has completely disappeared. It's still there, promise.

Remember: postpartum exercise is not about losing weight; the extra fat on your body is connected to your hormones and will pretty much not come off until it's not needed by your body or your baby anymore, particularly if you are breastfeeding. Yes,

* Pretty similar to the "common cold," but a man has it, so it appears to be fatal until it completely resolves in the normal amount of time.

some lucky bitches lose weight while breast-feeding, but the vast majority of mothers we know have a much different experience. You do not need to push yourself through pain and exhaustion to lose it. Instead, concentrate on healing and strengthening your body, because it has been through a lot.

SELF-CARE TOOLS YOU CAN BUY ON THE INTERNET THAT WILL MAKE YOUR RECOVERY MORE "LUXE"

- Fancy soft socks
- A nursing nightgown that makes you feel hot
- Korean skin care products
- A sleeping mask
- Bluetooth headphones (so you can watch TV/listen to tunes while endlessly breastfeeding without tangling your baby in cords)

There are many more tips to aid your postpartum recovery in the coming chapters, so be sure to read or skim through those *before* the baby is here and you have energy for precisely zero reading.

MENTAL HEALTH TRIAGE

Birth trauma is *real* and *common* and a legitimate reason to seek out care. It does not make you less of a warrior to admit that you have sustained injuries, whether they are physical or mental. Processing trauma when it happens is an important part of moving past it. Those amazing love hormones you feel toward your baby will sustain you for a while, but if there was a part of your birth experience that was awful or scary, *talk about it, write about it, and cry about it.* Tell someone you trust that you had a traumatic experience and need help. If they don't do anything to help you, tell someone else. Keep talking until someone listens and gets you to a trauma therapist, who will help you feel better. You deserve this, mama.

Very often, shame is the biggest barrier to getting mental health care. Shame tells us to isolate ourselves; that we are bad and cannot let anyone else know how terrible we are, or how terrible we feel. Women are raised to believe that motherhood will bring us ultimate fulfillment and peace and happiness. When it doesn't, we must be doing something wrong. Fortunately, this is pure bullshit. The truth is, hormones and lack of sleep make your brain do insane shit, and when it starts to do insane shit, you need to tell a professional so that they can help you get back to your normal brain chemicals.

Here are some dark thoughts that we've had in early motherhood and felt shame about, just in case you've had them too and need to know you're not a loveless monster mom:

- "I wish I hadn't had a baby; I miss my old life."
- "I thought this was supposed to be fun."
- "I wish I could run away."
- "Maybe I'm just crazy now, permanently?"
- "I'm a bad mother."
- "I'm a bad wife."
- "My family would be better off without me."

If any of these resonate with you, please know that you are deserving of love and help and you do not have to feel like this anymore, so tell someone. For more on the signs of postpartum depression, see page 203.

It's common for women to downplay our pain and wait too long to get help. Now's a great time to stop doing that. It is not selfish, because your baby deserves the happiest you. And if you're worried that maybe you're just a little sad, go to therapy anyway. It can't hurt.

Almost everyone needs therapy at some point, because life is hard and having an impartial guide to help you process it is invaluable. There is no population more deserving of this sort of care than new mothers, who are balancing challenging and exciting new stressors, dealing with emotionally disastrous hormone fluctuations, sleep deprivation, and marital conflict. It's all a natural part of becoming a family, but it can feel pretty heavy if you don't have someone to unload onto who isn't directly in the shit with you. Supportive partners are important, but complaining about your partner to your partner is usually just called a fight, not therapy.

Get a therapist, read self-help books that speak to your goals, use YouTube meditation videos to help you de-stress and process, write in a journal, set small and well-contained fires, get back on your meds; whatever mental health maintenance feels like for you, that's the right thing to do.

Tell your ob-gyn or midwife that you're struggling emotionally, if they're willing to listen, but they are not always the best place to go if you're really in trouble or need to go on meds. If they feel you're in immediate danger, they may refer you to the ER or psych ward, which in some cases is necessary but in other cases may just retraumatize you and keep you from your baby during an already stressful time. If you're stable, get a referral to a therapist or psychiatrist before you start to unload everything. Either way, make sure someone in your life knows how you're feeling and is actively helping you to get help.

FIND YOUR COMMUNITY

Many years ago, there was an interesting study[4] on the roots of addiction. Laboratory mice were given a choice between a normal water bottle and a water bottle laced with cocaine. The mice who had access to a community of other mice chose to drink the regular water, while the lonely mice drank the cocaine water until they eventually died. Our point is simple: if you have mom friends, you won't want to drink cocaine water, even if you are very tired, because they will also be very tired and understand that you are tired and you will not want to die.

Unfortunately, having a community in modern times is not as easy as it sounds. It's pretty unlikely that you're living in a close-knit group of families who are all having babies at the same time, unless you are in a cult. (Please stop reading and call 911! Leave the cult!) It's weirdly hard to make new friends as a grown-up, so again, prepare yourself by taking a prenatal yoga class, birthing class, or some other social gathering where you can get to know some randos who are gonna spit out a baby around the same time as you. It doesn't matter if you are similar people, as long as you get along. Having mom friends with babies who are the same age makes it much easier to socialize in the early days, as their nap times are more likely to line up. This is much more important than it sounds now; incompatible naps can hold you hostage and make you forget what it feels like to talk to another adult woman.

If you're an introvert who hates social gatherings, we are here to say: We see you. You matter, #twinsies. Find a group of moms on social media who you can chat with about diaper rash and how much sleep regressions suck. Not all mom groups are created equal, so be the creepy lurker in some different groups, and find some people who speak your language so you can curse with them sometimes. It helps. For more on mom friends, see "Building Your Crew and Keeping Your Sanity," page 243.

NOPE, YOU DON'T HAVE TO LET THEM VISIT

Maybe you truly welcome the visits of your supportive, respectful family. But if the thought of having to look another person in the eye when you just gave birth makes you ill, or you have a complicated or toxic dynamic, set some boundaries with friends and family. For example, no visits at the hospital, or no visits for x number of days, or no visits unless you do a load of laundry and make me an omelet. You probably know in your gut if you want certain people around, so find the courage to tell them what you need *before* the baby arrives.

Some people will take advantage of your exhaustion, badgering you to let them come see the baby and "help." Then they'll talk your ear off through that precious nap time, tell you about their own problems, leave you with some extra dirty dishes, and make you consider murder/suicide. Prepare those people now. In customer service, it's called "managing expectations." You can always cave and let them come at the last minute, but at least then you'll be overdelivering on your promise, instead of having to deal with some pushy person's disappointment when you are way too tired to argue. Here are some ways to tell them what's what:

- "Sorry, we're not going to have visitors for the first two weeks. The doctor says we should protect the baby from germs."*

- "Sorry, I won't be on my phone much, so I might not see your texts right away."

- "Sorry, I'm not feeling very well."†

- "Sorry, you're a very draining person to be around and we're not up for it right now."

This might require a careful setting of boundaries and resetting of boundaries with family members who don't respect them, but if you need some time to catch your breath after this baby comes, go ahead

---

* Using a doctor or expert as your excuse is a great way to pass along responsibility and defend yourself against attack.

† Maybe you don't have a cold, but think about it—a baby just ripped through you. Are you feeling well? No. Not amazing. Just because you have a perfect new baby who everyone wants to meet doesn't mean you have to hide the fact that you feel like shit.

and say it. Stick to your guns. Even if you have to say it again and again and again, chances are the person who's not respecting your request in the first place is not someone you want to have around disrespecting your requests when you're barely keeping your head above water with a newborn baby. This is your baby, your life, end of story.

Make sure your partner is supporting you in setting those boundaries. You may have to coach them in advance. This is new to them and they've probably never seen you in such a vulnerable state. Get on the same page so they can have your back when anyone tries to thwart your plans.

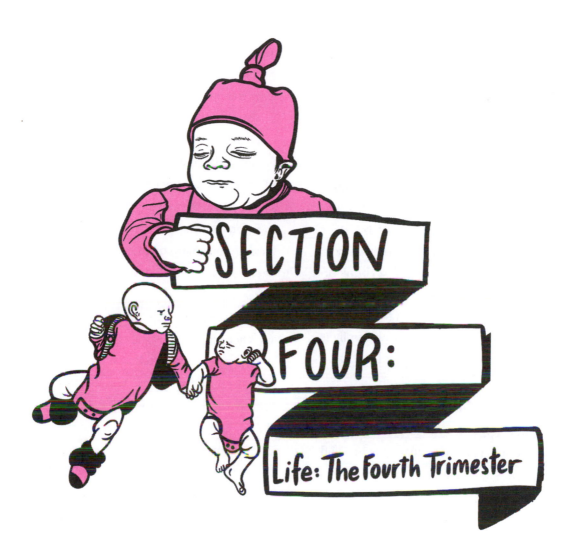

SECTION

FOUR:

Life: The Fourth Trimester

BABIES, THEY'RE JUST LIKE US!

Living with a baby is a bit like living with a celebrity. From the outside, babies seem exciting and fun and everyone wants to hear what it's like to be close to one. But behind the scenes they're very high-maintenance and not nearly as exciting as people think. Yes, your kin is a perfect precious bundle of joy, but early on they're mostly focused on getting milk drunk and flipping the fuck out at exhaustingly frequent intervals. In the fourth trimester, no one in your family is going to be living their best life.

Your tiny human is just as unpredictable as a full-size human. You'll comb the internet for solutions, but unfortunately your child is a unique snowflake of desperate and quickly changing needs! When you want them to be "good," remember that, like a downward spiraling celebrity, this little person has very little control over her own limbs or bowels and is just kind of a mess right now.

Babies are annoying by design. Scientists have actually learned that newborns consume every shred of your energy so that you're less likely to have sex and get pregnant with another baby, who might divide your attention and threaten their survival. At least you don't have two babies?*

Every parent feels like they have no idea what they're doing. You'll live a million tiny failures a day, but some will really stand out. At some point every parent makes a mistake so huge that they think, "Oh my God, I am the worst mother on earth!" This might be locking your baby in the car, walking their head into a doorway, or *letting your baby fall off the bed.*

You'll feel horrible. You'll be ashamed. But then slowly other parents will come out of the woodwork to tell you that they also once dropped their baby. Actually, *their* baby fell off the bed THREE TIMES. And you'll think, "Now *that* sounds dangerous. I've dropped my baby only once! Look at me! I'm an *amazing* parent!" Over time, you'll learn that babies are sturdier than they look. And they are sturdy by design because new parents are incredibly tired. By the time you learn what not to do, it's too late. Here are some . . .

---

* Sorry, parents of twins! None of us know how you suffer.

LESSONS YOU WON'T LEARN UNTIL YOU HAVE A SECOND CHILD EVEN THOUGH YOU'RE READING THEM NOW

Don't Jump at Every Gurgle

They are not dying. They just have weird tiny little mouths and tiny throats and they're still bringing up some uterus juice from their teeny lungs. They will sound like they're on the brink of death, but they are just tiny gurgly tricksters who want every second of your attention.

Babies Just Are Fussy

Maybe someone somewhere had a baby who never produced gas or got overtired or hungry, but most of the time babies will just be babies, which means they'll cry and cry and cry. Someday when you're old and not talking sense anymore, you'll go up to a screaming baby and say, "I miss those little cries," like a total lunatic.

All They Want Is You

Your baby is like a parasite trying to stay attached to you. This won't last forever, so for now, be glad they're happy being snuggled against you and aren't asking you to buy them an iPhone. You are enough.

While it's annoying to have someone on you all day long, it's also sort of cool to have someone be so ecstatic to see you even if you just left the room for two seconds to reheat your coffee. You get to introduce this cool little person to the whole wide world, teaching them what grass is, how food tastes, and how to laugh at the dumbest things. It will get more fun as you go along.

Everything Will Forever Be Covered in Stains Until Your Whole Life Is a Stain

It's spit-up and poop, then baby food and eventually the great outdoors. It will be all over everything, until one day your old idea of "dirty" becomes your new "Wow, I wish I could live *there*." Consider this shock therapy for any OCD tendencies you have.

This is a magically consuming time you are living in. And it'll be over before you know it, or at least it will seem like that when it's over, because your brain is too exhausted now to form coherent memories. Beware the advice and opinions of people who had a baby more than a year ago. If they think there is an easy solve for any of this, they are remembering wrong. They're remembering their chubby six-month-old while you're over here with a smushy little one-month-old. If they say anything other than "I don't miss that age," they are wrong. Their words are lies.

But remember—it gets better. Because almost anything is better than being a sleepless prisoner in your own home. And in the end, you made a person! You're amazing!

Why Is My Baby Crying?

Your baby could be crying for any of the reasons below, but it may not be any of them at all.

- Hungry
- Tired
- Gas
- Wet diaper (in our experience most babies actually DGAF if they are wet)
- Wants you to hold them
- Doesn't want to be held
- Wants to be jiggled in a very specific way for two hours straight
- Just feeling weird today
- You wouldn't get it!

Why Do I Feel Nuts When My Baby Cries?

Just as you're finally about to drift off into exhausted sleep, inevitably, it happens: Your baby wakes up and starts to cry. Your partner stays snoring peacefully next to you, but suddenly you've got a racing heart and hyperfocus. Must. Help. Baby. Again.

You're not nuts, but man, it sure can feel like it. What's to blame? As usual, hormones. Oxytocin, to be exact. That crazy love hormone that helps you bond with your baby and triggers letdown of milk to feed your baby is also responsible for how nuts you feel when she cries.

When your baby cries, your brain releases oxytocin into its left auditory complex, allowing you to become superhero-level attuned to your baby's cry of distress. Not only that, but your brain is literally changing to help you meet your baby's needs. There's not really anything you can do about it, but maybe you feel a little less crazy now after reading this? Since your partner doesn't have this chemical reaction happening in them, they'll need a little help fine-tuning this parental reflex. Might we recommend a swift pillow to the head each time the baby cries and they don't wake up?

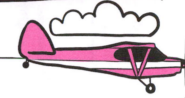

DOES MY BABY HAVE COLIC...

OR IS HE JUST AN ASSHOLE?

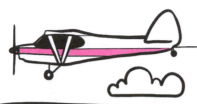

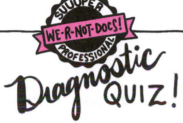

SUUUPER · WE·R·NOT·DOCS! · PROFESSIONAL

Diagnostic QUIZ!

1. HOW MUCH DOES YOUR BABY CRY?

A) A LOT.

B) MORE THAN THREE HOURS IN A ROW, AT LEAST THREE DAYS A WEEK, FOR AT LEAST THREE WEEKS, EVEN THOUGH THEY SEEM OTHERWISE HEALTHY.

FLIP THE BOOK FOR ANSWERS!

ANSWER KEY:

IF YOU ANSWERED A:

YOU HAVE A NORMAL ASSHOLE BABY.

IF YOU ANSWERED B:

SORRY, IT SOUNDS LIKE YOUR BABY HAS COLIC. SOME THINGS THAT MIGHT HELP ARE: WEARING YOUR BABY AT ALL TIMES (SO YOU CAN HEAR THEIR SCREAMING UP CLOSE), GETTING A SHUSHER (A LITTLE WHITE NOISE MACHINE THAT IS MEANT TO SOOTHE YOUR BABY OR AT LEAST SLIGHTLY DROWN OUT THEIR CRIES), AND LEAVING YOUR BABY FOR AS LONG AS YOU CAN POSSIBLY STOMACH/AFFORD. SERIOUSLY, TAKE CARE OF YOURSELF. COLIC IS TRULY INSANE.

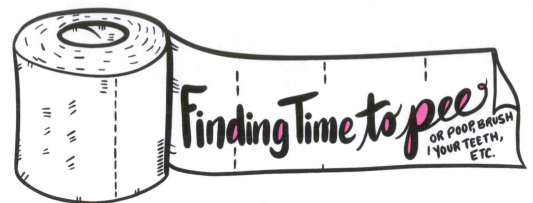

Finding Time to pee
OR POOP, BRUSH YOUR TEETH, ETC.

In attempting to meet all of your baby's needs, it will become very difficult to find time to pee. The chart below illustrates just how difficult this will now be:

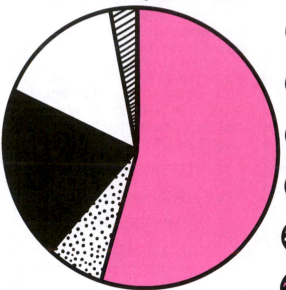

- ⬤ Time spent feeding the baby
- ⬤ Time spent burping the baby
- ⬤ Time spent jiggling the baby to sleep
- ◯ Time spent checking to make sure the baby is breathing
- ⬤ Time spent sleeping
- ⬤ Time left for peeing (0%)

THERE'S NO WRONG WAY TO FEED A BABY

> Don't know how you feel about milking your boobs? In this chapter, we'll discuss some of the pros and cons of breastfeeding and formula. There is not a wrong decision here, so long as your baby is getting the nutrition she needs.

If you're breastfeeding there will be a couple of days before your milk comes in when your boobs produce only a yellow substance called colostrum. During this time, all available medical professionals will gather to inform you of how urgent it is for your baby to have milk, as if you are intentionally withholding it. Your baby, who is also eager for the milk, will try to inform your body of what it's supposed to be doing, the only way he or she knows how—by sucking your tender nips round the clock and ensuring that your broken body has not a moment to rest and repair. You'll probably be so tired and sore, from your nips to freshly popped vagina (or C-section scar) that you'll want to die. But you'll decide to stay alive for the sake of your baby.

While it's important to have your baby nursing as often as possible to encourage your milk to come in, sometimes there are medical issues, or the stress of low supply is too hard on the mother and/or baby. It's okay to give your baby formula, even if you're attempting to breastfeed. Talk to your providers about how you and your baby are doing in order to make an informed decision.

What's most important is that your baby regains her birth weight[*] and grows at a healthy rate.

DID YOU FRIGGIN' KNOW?

Colostrum (the yellow substance coming out of your nipples before your milk comes in) is referred to as "liquid gold" because it is filled with antibodies and all babies who get these antibodies grow up to be incredibly wealthy and successful while the babies who don't get it end up on reality shows at best.

---

[*] Babies often lose a small percentage of their birth weight in the first week (slightly more if they're breastfed), but they should regain it in the second week.

BREASTFEEDING
—OR—
FORMULA
—OR—
BOTH?!

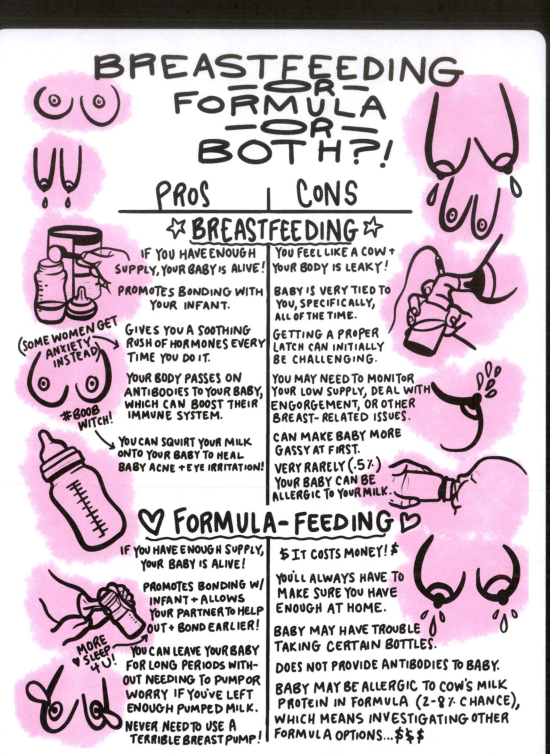

PROS	CONS

☆ BREASTFEEDING ☆

PROS	CONS
IF YOU HAVE ENOUGH SUPPLY, YOUR BABY IS ALIVE!	YOU FEEL LIKE A COW + YOUR BODY IS LEAKY!
PROMOTES BONDING WITH YOUR INFANT.	BABY IS VERY TIED TO YOU, SPECIFICALLY, ALL OF THE TIME.
GIVES YOU A SOOTHING RUSH OF HORMONES EVERY TIME YOU DO IT.	GETTING A PROPER LATCH CAN INITIALLY BE CHALLENGING.
YOUR BODY PASSES ON ANTIBODIES TO YOUR BABY, WHICH CAN BOOST THEIR IMMUNE SYSTEM.	YOU MAY NEED TO MONITOR YOUR LOW SUPPLY, DEAL WITH ENGORGEMENT, OR OTHER BREAST-RELATED ISSUES.
YOU CAN SQUIRT YOUR MILK ONTO YOUR BABY TO HEAL BABY ACNE + EYE IRRITATION!	CAN MAKE BABY MORE GASSY AT FIRST.
	VERY RARELY (.5%) YOUR BABY CAN BE ALLERGIC TO YOUR MILK.

(SOME WOMEN GET ANXIETY INSTEAD)

#BOOB WITCH!

♡ FORMULA-FEEDING ♡

PROS	CONS
IF YOU HAVE ENOUGH SUPPLY, YOUR BABY IS ALIVE!	$ IT COSTS MONEY! $
PROMOTES BONDING W/ INFANT + ALLOWS YOUR PARTNER TO HELP OUT + BOND EARLIER!	YOU'LL ALWAYS HAVE TO MAKE SURE YOU HAVE ENOUGH AT HOME.
YOU CAN LEAVE YOUR BABY FOR LONG PERIODS WITH-OUT NEEDING TO PUMP OR WORRY IF YOU'VE LEFT ENOUGH PUMPED MILK.	BABY MAY HAVE TROUBLE TAKING CERTAIN BOTTLES.
NEVER NEED TO USE A TERRIBLE BREAST PUMP!	DOES NOT PROVIDE ANTIBODIES TO BABY.
	BABY MAY BE ALLERGIC TO COW'S MILK PROTEIN IN FORMULA (2-8% CHANCE), WHICH MEANS INVESTIGATING OTHER FORMULA OPTIONS...$$$

MORE SLEEP 4 U!

Jaundice

Bilirubin (pronounced "billy-rube-in," like the name of a fictional talking bear) is a yellow substance produced when the body breaks down blood cells. Since newborns are often born with excess blood cells and their liver's waste-disposal system is still maturing, their skin may develop a yellowish color known as **jaundice**. Increasing bilirubin levels could eventually damage your baby's brain, so they'll be tested at the hospital, and sometimes after you leave, to make sure your baby's bilirubin levels are falling.

Feeding your baby as often as possible helps bilirubin levels fall since this encourages their body to eliminate waste. Bilirubin is generally more of an issue for breastfed babies since their mother's milk may take time to come in. This is why it's important to find a good latch, and if necessary supplement with formula. Even if your baby's bilirubin levels aren't falling, the jaundice can be treated fairly easily by placing your baby under phototherapy lights or a bilirubin blanket, which will dissolve the bilirubin.

In cases of prolonged jaundice, the mother's breast milk sometimes contains a substance that interferes with bilirubin absorption. Therefore the doctor may recommend pumping while feeding with baby formula until the condition clears.

Poop Logs and Feeding Charts

To ensure your baby is getting enough milk, your provider may ask you to make a record of when they fed, peed, and pooped. You will do this round the clock and in the dead of night, so it should look something like the example on the next page.

Pee diaper	Poop diaper	Feeding ♡

MONDAY ♡   4AM

6AM → VERY green (NORMAL?? Call ped??)

She said fine, sounded annoyed? *Research new pediatrician.*

4AM → 20 MINS EACH BOOB ♡

→ 7AM

(JUST A LITTLE WET, HOW WET IS TOO WET? GOOGLE THIS LATER B/C DIAPERS ARE $$$)

8AM → BLOWOUT IN STROLLER ON MORNING WALK. (STILL GREEN...ISH.)

6AM → breakfast (6oz.) bottle with Dad ♡

6:30AM → 20 MINS EACH BOOB AGAIN?

POSSIBLE GROWTH SPURT?

9AM

11:30AM → POST-BOTTLE SHIT-STORM TO MAKE ROOM FOR DESSERT. ↑ BOOBS.

9AM – 11AM NURSE TO SLEEP 4 FIRST NAP BUT WON'T UNLATCH SO I GUESS I WILL LAY HERE?

11AM

~~TUESDAY~~ (NEVER MIND, MONDAY CONT.)

WHY ARE DAYS SO LONG NOW?!

HE PEES PLENTY. IT'S FINE.

(LOOKS LIKE FANCY MUSTARD?)

I AM STARVING.

12:30 → MORE MUSTARD SHIT. WAITING 4 AMAZON DIAPER DELIVERY + HOLDING BABY OVER TOILET...

11:30AM → LUNCH BOTTLE WITH DESSERT BOOBS?

THE FUCK IS MY LIFE NOW?

STILL MONDAY → LOST CHART FOR SEVERAL HOURS UNDER PILE OF LAUNDRY...

HE PEED IN MY FACE 3X BUT **NEVER** IN DIAPER.

LOST COUNT, BABY SHIT IN SWING + IN MY FUCKING BED

6:45PM PAJAMA BLOWOUT AS SOON AS BABY IS ASLEEP.

CONSTANT FEEDING UNTIL 5:30 PM WHEN HUSBAND CAME HOME, NOW HIDING IN BATHROOM CRYING OVER DESTROYED NIPPLES.

BEDTIME BOTTLE (8 OZ.) @ 6:30PM

30 MINS. EACH BOOB TO SOOTHE BACK 2 SLEEP

FINALLY ASLEEP "FOR THE NIGHT."

4AM HE DEFINITELY SHIT IN HIS SLEEP BUT THERE'S NO FUCKING

11PM → 15 MINS EACH BOOB
2 AM → " " "
3:15AM → " " " "
" " " "
" " " " !!!

OH, *THAT'S* WHAT THESE BOOBS ARE FOR! A GUIDE TO BREASTFEEDING

> Breastfeeding is a beautiful, natural way to get your boobs smashed to smithereens. It has amazing health benefits as well as many hilariously messy aspects. When your breast milk first comes in, it can be grueling. Not only are your boobs in pain, but you'll feel crazed due to fluctuating oxytocin levels and the difficulty of getting your baby to latch in a way that doesn't feel like she's trying to sever your nipples from your body.

ESSENTIAL TIPS FOR SUCCESS

Look for the Boob Helpers

It's very common to have trouble breastfeeding early on. You may be dealing with inverted nipples, your baby's tongue-tie, or maybe the baby-to-boob situation just doesn't come as intuitively as you'd hoped. Many women need help getting to the bottom of breastfeeding woes. Online videos can help you understand latch, or you might be able to find a lactation consultant covered by your health insurance. La Leche League holds free meetings for breastfeeding moms to share support and information.

Breastfeeding resources can be a great help, but they can sometimes make women feel pressured or shamed for unavoidable difficulties. If you're struggling with milk supply, painful latch, or any other issue that makes breastfeeding a stress on your mental health or your baby's health, it's okay to supplement with formula or stop breastfeeding altogether. Don't listen to anyone who makes you feel ashamed.

Drink *All* the Water

In the beginning, there will be thirst, and it will be unquenchable. Put a large pitcher of water next to your bed, since you won't want to interrupt the delicate process of trying to situate a baby on your boob without her falling off your nipple. Actually, you know those beer helmets frat boys wear? Load up one with two cans of Pamplemousse La Croix and you've got hands-free hydration, baby!

Try Different Breastfeeding Holds

There are a surprisingly wide variety of ways to hold your baby while you breastfeed. The classic positions like the cross-

(continued on page 179)

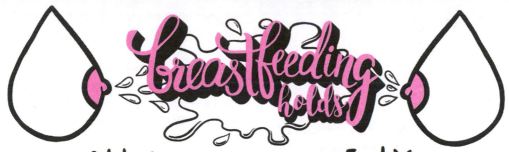

Breastfeeding holds

FOOTBALL HOLD

SIDE-LYING

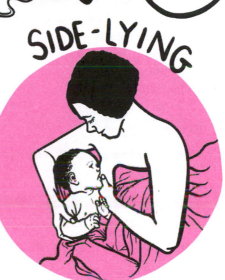

CROSS-CRADLE HOLD

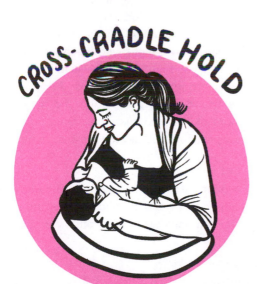

LYING BACK

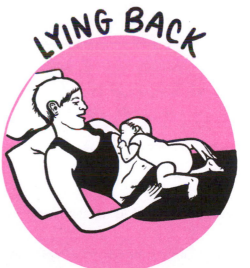

A Guide to Engorgement

Engorgement is a normal and terribly unpleasant thing that happens about two to five days after birth, when your milk comes in. Your breasts are like, "Uhhh, whaaaat? We are filling with fluid?!" As if they haven't had nine months to prepare for this like the rest of us. Engorgement rarely lasts more than twenty-four hours, thank God.

Side effects include:

* Breasts of stone

* Hot boobz (not in a sexy way, just very warm to the touch)

* Shiny and tight bodybuilder skin, but only on your boobs

* Low-grade fever of approximately 100

* Flat nipples that make latching difficult

* Rage

HOW TO PREVENT IT

While you can't really avoid it when your milk comes in, you can help it not come back by following some rules.

Nurse Often

Nurse your baby on their cue, which you will get to know pretty quickly. (Don't listen to your part-ner when they tell you that the baby is hungry though; that just means they don't want to change a diaper.) Aim to nurse your baby ten times in a twenty-four-hour period, and try not to skip feedings, especially in the early days when it's really easy for your boobs to fill up in a few hours. Don't want to wake a sleeping baby? Us either; pump that shit!

Empty Those Puppies

If your baby falls asleep on your boob, turning her around to nurse on the other side will generally rouse her enough to nurse again, and then when she's done with boob two she will definitely be passed the F out enough to put down. Your baby often signals when she's fully drained one boob by abruptly coming off the breast, or biting you for seemingly no reason. Try to empty one boob before switching, since your baby gets a different quality of milk as she's chugging along. When he first starts feeding, he gets the foremilk, which is sweeter and encourages him to keep going. Eventually, your letdown* is triggered and she'll get the hindmilk, which is fattier, keeps her fuller longer, gaining more weight, and feeling less gassy. You may find that your baby is full before the second boob is fully emptied. Just start the next feeding on that boob† and they'll get more of the hindmilk. Over time, your milk supply should adjust to your baby's needs.

Get a Good Latch

A good latch will help your baby efficiently empty your boobs; a bad latch will ruin your life. You don't wanna just stick your boob in

---

* Letdown (n): when the milk in your boobs is like "Let me out of here!"

† Some women will clip something to their bra strap to remember which side they left off on.

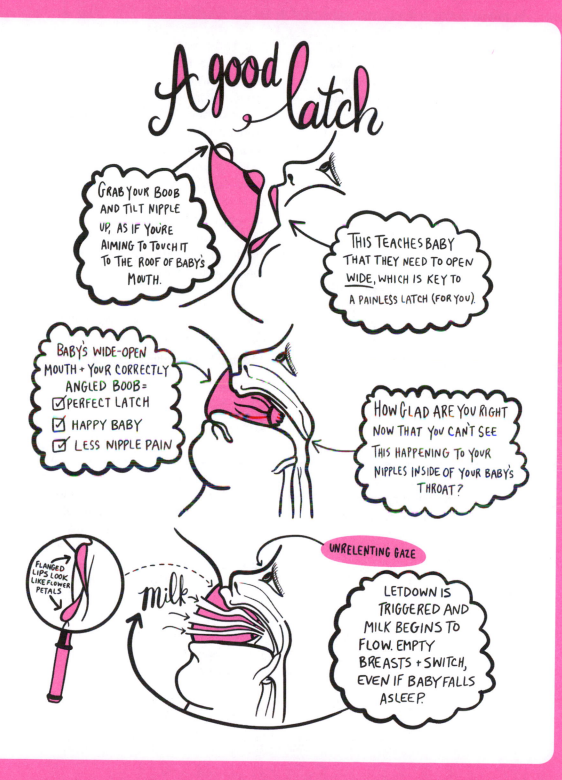

your baby's mouth. At least not while you're both getting the hang of things. The key to sustainably breastfeeding is doing it in a way where you don't feel like your boobs are being sawn off. This means getting your boob deep into the baby's mouth so they're not gnawing on the nipple. You'll want to squeeze your breast and tilt your nipple up toward the roof of the baby's mouth as you insert it into their mouth. After a while you won't have to think so much about what you're doing.

Pump It UP!

If you have an abundant supply and a sleepy AF baby, pump! But don't pump too much. The goal is to pump until you're comfortable, but not increase your milk supply (unless for some reason you *are* trying to increase supply, for example, if you're nursing twins). Your boobs are very smart and sexy computers, and they're learning how much milk to make. A pump can make them think you have a very hungry baby, if you're not careful and intentional about how much you're pumping. If you have a *lot* of milk, consider donating it to a milk bank for mamas who need some help with their supply.

HOW TO TREAT IT

If you end up engorged, it's okay! We can fix this! Here's what to do.

Before a Feeding

Massage your breasts (toward the nipple, as if you're milking a cow, which you pretty much are) and your entire chest wall before your baby eats. You can also apply cold compresses for about twenty minutes beforehand, which will help with the inflammation and pain.

If your baby is having trouble latching on to your flat, hard nipples, jump in the shower beforehand. *Do not* let the hot water run directly on your tits; that will hurt a lot. Instead, let the warm water soothe your back muscles and relax you as you gently hand-express some milk from your nipples in order to trigger letdown and relieve some of the tightness, which will make it easier for your baby to latch.

Between Feedings

Take the edge off by pumping a little bit, or hand-expressing only until you feel comfortable again. This will avoid overproduction.

Cabbage Leaves
(Yes, That Thing You Heard Is True)

Speaking of overproduction (you busy little worker bee, you) if you have too much milk, cabbage leaves can help! Like many ingenious cures for the female body developed by wise women out of necessity (and a complete lack of interest from the medical community), cabbage leaves are a very effective way to reduce your milk supply. Wash the cabbage leaves, obviously, and chill them in the fridge for added relief. Stuff them leaves in your bra for about twenty minutes before a feeding, but don't do this more than three times a day, or you may decrease supply too much. Stop once you no longer have an oversupply.

cradle hold are good for monitoring your baby while you figure out your latch, but as the baby gets bigger you can play around. Side-lying is a nice way to breastfeed if you're cosleeping and don't want to wake up too much in the night to breastfeed, though it can be hard to maneuver when the baby is still very small. Both side-lying and the football hold can help keep the baby's weight off your abdomen if you're recovering from a C-section. The lying-back pose can also make it a bit harder to get your baby to latch but does make you look super chill and cool.

Master the Boob-to-Pacifier Switcheroo

Once your baby passes out on top of you, you'll want to do other things, like go to the bathroom or eat food. But if you pull them off the boob (unless they've got that milk-drunk, totally dead face going on), they want immediately back on. This is where you must master the pacifier switcheroo. It takes some practice to pull off this daring heist, but you'll perfect the technique of quickly replacing your nipple with a pacifier. Some babies will spot the dupe right way, but over time they should learn to be okay with a paci instead of 24-7 boob, and you'll be able to wear a shirt sometimes.

Treating Plugged Ducts

Occasionally, one of your milk ducts gets obstructed, and the area becomes swollen and inflamed. If you notice local tenderness in the area, try soaking in an Epsom salt bath (or just hold your boob in a bowl full of Epsom-salt water, if you're short on time) and nurse immediately afterward. Do not avoid nursing on this side; feeding your baby is actually the most effective way to clear the milk duct and solve the problem.

Having a "Food" Boob Is Okay

Often one boob is a better producer than the other. You may even find that over time, your baby prefers this boob. This is normal and fine. Sure, you may have wildly different-size boobs, but it's nothing to worry about.

Breastfeeding Can Make You Feel Amazing

Like birth, breastfeeding releases oxytocin. This is the hormone we associate with love and sex and everything nice. So sitting down to breastfeed may make you feel relaxed. This is nature's way of encouraging you to bond with your baby, and it can be a source of real joy. You may find that when you're overdue for a feeding you can get a bit cranky as your body is craving this release.

Breastfeeding Can Make You Feel Awful

Some women have a very different reaction to breastfeeding, and this is also normal. These women can experience anxiety during letdown, kinda like your body is like, "Nope this sucks, let's run!" Take some deep breaths and make sure you're sitting comfortably and nothing is causing you to feel pain, like a bad latch or a lumpy couch. If necessary, stop and find a more comfortable spot to feed, and you may be able to calm your nervous system down a little more.

DID YOU FRIGGIN' KNOW?

Boob Spray

If you're breastfeeding, your boobs will probably leak. And when you take off a tight bra and unleash those beauts, nipples swaying in the cool air like a porn scene that's about to get weird, the milk will spurt like a whale's blowhole and the clean towel you grabbed for your shower will be covered in milk, just like everything else you own.

BREASTFEEDING ACCOUTREMENTS

You'd think your boobs would be all you need, and mostly they are, but it really takes a village of ridiculous products to try to breastfeed in the modern world.

Breastfeeding Pillows

It takes a lot of effort to get little baby bodies perched up near your boob at the right angle. As they get bigger, they can kind of just flop onto you. But in the beginning they have no size or strength, so despite how light they are, it takes more effort to hold them where they need to be. This is where breastfeeding pillows come in. There are many on the market, and you may need to supplement with additional pillows to give yourself a sort of pillow throne to support your aching arms.

Nursing Bras

In the first few weeks you can chill out at home braless, but eventually you've gotta get nursing bras. Trying to nurse with a regular bra on is pretty infuriating, as the bra keeps shifting up toward your nipple, causing the baby to come unlatched, with milk spraying everywhere. A supportive nursing bra will also help compress your boobs so they're not rubbing against your shirt and thinking it's time to do their thing and spray. So stock up on some big, ugly mom-bras. Make sure you find the right size, since your prepregnancy size will not accommodate you. Make sure your titty-sling is comfortable, well fitting, and supportive. Anything else puts you at risk for plugged ducts, mastitis, and becoming physically violent with strangers.

MASTITIS—WUZZAT?

If you have mastitis, you'll know. Your breasts will be red and painful, and you will have a temperature over 100.6 and flulike symptoms such as chills and body aches. You will feel like shit and have horrible fire boobs. If this happens, call your provider immediately.

Button-down Shirts

You don't necessarily need fancy nursing shirts (though if you find some good ones, cool!). Any shirt that opens in the front will be a lifesaver, especially if you don't love stretching the neck of your shirts out, or exposing your post-baby belly to everyone when you lift it up. Some women layer a T-shirt over a tank top, so they can lift up the top layer, avoiding the aforementioned belly display, while camouflaging the visible boob situation with the top layer.

Breast Pads

If you're alone at home, you can shove a sock in your bra. But if you have to be out in the world, and goddess forbid at work, you don't want big leaky stains peering from the top of your shirt like the eyes of a cartoon character. Breast pads help absorb leaks. Some of us have to change them way more often than others.

HOW TO OPENLY BREASTFEED (WHILE COVERED)

Before you're confronted with reality, you might plan on being the perfect beautiful mom—one who hasn't given up, has a gel mani, and erases breastfeeding stigmas by plopping out her full breasts in any room. But when you're sleepless, hormonal, and unshowered, you're not always in the mood to bare it all. And you don't always want to introduce your boss, father-in-law, brother, or mechanic to the exact size, shape, and color of your nipples.

If you don't give a fuck, go for it! But it's okay to not want to watch other people watch your boobs. Throw a burp cloth on there or buy a nursing cover, which will allow you to see your baby while keeping the cloth out of her way. Some babies friggin' hate having anything near their face and can't breastfeed with a cover, which means you either have to embrace the DGAF breastfeeding lifestyle or always find a private spot. Both present awkward challenges, and either might be preferable depending on how you feel, where you are, and who is trying to spy your boobs. We support whatever you choose, wherever and whenever.

HOW TO NONCHALANTLY SQUEEZE YOUR BOOBS TO CHECK THEIR FULLNESS

You'll likely need to constantly gauge how soon you should feed based on how starving your baby seems and how overflowing your boobs feel. Sometimes they'll become engorged and start to hurt, and you need to empty the tank. This prevents you from getting a clogged duct, mastitis, or just leaking all over yourself while you try to have a normal conversation. You'll be able to tell how full you are by the firmness of your boobs. Your partner will get used to the sight of you feeling yourself, but out in public, you'll need to learn covert methods. Maybe the casual neck scratch into resting your hand on your chest?

WHEN YOU'RE FEELING *VERY* DONE WITH BREASTFEEDING

Breastfeeding is sometimes great and healthy and awesome and empowering, and some-times it's not. It might be that your baby has an allergy that is making her sick, you're not making enough milk, your breasts hurt so badly that you want to die, your supply is dwindling, breastfeeding is making you upset or unstable, or it's just been too fucking long. Whatever the reason, if breastfeeding is not working for your family, that is okay. The best kind of baby is a fed baby, and the best kind of mama is a not-suffering mama.

Weaning Before You Planned To

Weaning before you or your baby is ready can be intense, and not just because it's another huge hormonal shift for you. Also: other people. Other people loooove to have opinions about your tits, especially men people and old-lady people. Sometimes these people will try to convince you to "keep going, because it gets easier," and these people can fuck right off. Other people will tell you that you should definitely stop but not tell you how to stop, just that you should. These people can fuck right off too; ask them if they're willing to come over at 3:00 a.m. and help you not breastfeed your screaming baby.

The truth is: it is literally no one else's business how you feed your baby, and only you know what is best for the both of you.

You Can Eat Even More Now!

One of the rare perks of breastfeeding is eating more food. You may have thought your eating days were over now that there isn't a person in you, but now you're actually nourishing an even bigger person with your body. You may or may not lose weight while breastfeeding, but either way, you're feeding a baby with your body and need to make sure you get adequate nutrition, which is fun!

Here are some things that will boost milk supply:

* **Water.** We said it before, but we'll say it again. It's hard to fathom just how much water your body needs now. Drink all of it.

* **Oats.** You can get oats in the form of oatmeal, oatmeal cookies, or even certain kinds of beer! Just don't drink too much alcohol right before you breastfeed/pump.

* **Barley.** If you keep barley around the house, great. If you don't, maybe have a stout. Just keep an eye on the results. Alcohol can decrease milk supply.

* **A bunch of other roots/berries/seeds/etc.** Just like when you were pregnant, the more closely your food resembles the actual thing that grew out of the ground or walked on the ground, the more likely it is that you're getting nutrients and not just processed garbage. So try to eat fresh, tasty things and it'll be better for you, your baby, and your taste buds.

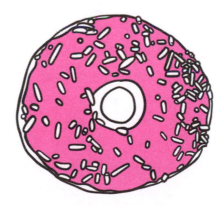

Night Weaning

At some point, children sleep through the night on their own, even if you do nothing to help them learn this skill. Some (fake) babies do it at six weeks, while other (most) children wake multiple times a night well into toddlerhood.

Somewhere between four to six months, your baby stops physically needing to eat in the middle of the night. Your pediatrician will usually give you the go-ahead to night wean, and you will say, "Oh, great! I guess I'll be sleeping through the night from now on!" Then he will drive home to his empty-nest doctor mansion and laugh and laugh, because no, you will not.

If you are really ready to stop breastfeeding at night, the best way to do this is by having your partner take over bedtime. Your baby will *hate this* at first, and she will scream and scream, and you will doubt yourself and wonder if you are a sociopath for trying this at all. You're not, you're just a very tired human woman. Put on some headphones and turn the music up real loud. Leave the house if you have to. Forbid your partner from texting you, or put your phone on airplane mode. *Remember: a baby crying in someone's arms is okay, even though your crazy hormones will tell your body that it's not okay and you need to save the crying baby immediately.*

Weaning for Good

Conceptually, the weaning process is pretty simple: start giving your baby other food and/or other milks, and eliminate breastfeeding sessions one by one until you're not breastfeeding anymore. Bedtime feeding is usually the last to go. If you're doing "baby-led weaning," you let the baby . . . lead . . . ? Otherwise you lead, probably? Sounds easy enough, right?

Unfortunately, babies don't usually go with the flow, and they're not super good at deciding what's best for the family. They are, however, *very* good at screaming at the top of their lungs and making you feel like you're going to have a heart attack until you put your boob in their mouth. This can muddy the process a bit.

In reality, weaning goes like this: Try to breastfeed less. Offer other things, with a slowly building desperation and lower and lower standards. Try about seven different bottles until you find one that is "very boob-like," and seems to work at least sometimes. Decide to try pacifiers again, even though she has never been interested. Let her play with your boobs inside of your shirt in public, rather than pull one out. Consider rubbing hot sauce on your nipples. Experiment with going out at bedtime and then get frantic texts from your partner and rush home and give in. Discover that if you just are constantly moving and engaging and keeping her busy, she doesn't ask. Then, when one of you gets sick or really tired, end up lying on the floor and breastfeeding for most of the afternoon.

Sometimes weaning is way easier than all this and babies just sort of slowly lose interest. But no matter when it happens, weaning is emotional. It signifies a really important (and positive!) physical and emotional shift for you and your baby: you are no longer their only source of comfort and sustenance. Sad about weaning? That's normal! Throw some money at that shit and buy a super-sappy piece of commemorative jewelry made from your breast milk. Then, for the rest of your life when someone says, "What kind of stone is that in your ring, opal?" you can stare deep into their eyes and hold their hands in yours and say, "No, that's my own milk. I had it preserved." People love that. They'll feel really comfortable around you after that.

THE NOT-FREEDOM OF BREAST PUMPING

Breastfeeding is hard enough as is, but you can also throw in some breast pumping for a fun way to get those nips pinched even when you're away from your baby. Hooray! Breast pumping is basically a necessity if you want to leave your breastfed baby for more than three or four hours without diminishing your milk supply.

How to Store Enough Milk to Feed a Small Infant Army

If you're exclusively breastfeeding, you can't just pump while you're away, you have to build up a supply to leave in the first place. This means pumpin' as much as possible between feedings, while also leaving enough for your baby's next feeding. If you're exclusively breastfeeding (not using any formula), you need to save up a lot. Your baby might chug more than usual in the stress of your absence, or a caregiver will heat up a bottle that the baby doesn't really want and it will spoil and go to waste. Once heated, breast milk needs to be used within a few hours because it goes bad very quickly. It cannot be put back in the fridge and reheated a second time. Make this very clear to caregivers lest your meticulous devotion to pumping goes down the drain.

Breast milk must be stored in the fridge or freezer. If stored in the fridge it will need to be used within a few days. It can last much longer in the freezer, though it may lose a tiny bit of nutritional value and will take longer to defrost. It's not recommended to microwave breast milk to defrost, because that could lower the nutritional quality of the milk even more, or make it too hot for your baby to drink. Somehow, even bottles and bottles stacked up in your freezer are not always enough to keep up with your baby. So get pumping.

The Ways You'll Fail at Your New Job as Breast-Pump Technician

Finding time to strap a milk machine to your breasts during the precious time you have away from your child is one of life's true miseries. Fortunately there's also a variety of ways for your mobile milking unit to go wrong, due to your sleep-deprived oversight:

- You forget to bring just one small part, which renders the entire forty-pound machine you've been hauling useless.

- You forget to connect bottles to the pump and end up pumping a bunch of milk into your lap.

- Just as you finish squeezing every last drop out of your sore boobs, your tired and overcaffeinated arm knocks the not-yet-sealed bottle over, reducing you to a pile of tears.

- You're too busy for one of your pumping sessions and now only have half the milk to show for the day.

- Your milk comes out like a geyser, and before you think to change the bottle, the milk starts overflowing all over you.

- The breast shield (the big suctiony milker part that goes on your boob) comes loose and has been fruitlessly milking the part of your boob next to your nipple for five minutes.

- You drag the milk all the way home and collapse on your couch, accidentally leaving it in your bag to go bad overnight.

Pumping is an annoying and constant interruption, but you can try to reframe it as a little break from the grind, a time to slow down away from your coworkers. If you can bear to stop multitasking, try to use this time to breathe and stare into space. As someone who's pumping all the livelong day, you deserve it, and your milk production will be better if you're not so amped.

PUMP HACKS

The pump life literally sucks, but here are ways to make things a bit easier:

Pump Early and Pump Often

Whether you're trying to build up a milk supply in advance of going back to work, or you're going to work later today, getting a pump session in early in the morning is helpful because it's when your supply is highest. Depending on supply, you may be able to pump some and still nurse your baby right after. Often your baby is better at fully emptying the breast than a machine (go, humans!). If you're not pumping as much milk as you'd like, try adding in another pumping session in between your others. As miserable as this sounds, over time, it may trigger your body to produce more milk.

Massage Your Breasts

Since you won't necessarily experience the same hormones that accompany the touch and smell of your little one, your body won't have as much of a natural letdown response, and you may need to help things along. You can massage before you pump and continue squeezing as you go. This is especially useful if you have a limited amount of time to pump.

Get a Hand Pump as a Backup

If you're on a plane, train, or somewhere you want to pump discreetly without the aggressive stares of everyone around you, a hand pump is much quieter. It's also smaller and easier to carry around than a mechanical pump. You will definitely want the real-deal electric pump for multiple-times-per-day pumping. But if you forget a part or battery or your whole pump altogether, hand pumps are relatively cheap and can often be found at drugstores, so you don't have to make the trek to a baby superstore.

Buy Double the Pump Parts

If you can afford it, two sets of pump parts allow you to throw one in the dishwasher and still have a clean set in the morning as you're rushing off to work.

Microwave Parts to Save Time

There are bags and plastic containers you can buy that sterilize your pump parts in the microwave when you don't have time to fully wash them (rinse off the milk before you do this).

Invest in a Good Storage Bag

You'll want something easy to carry, whether it's the bag your pump comes in or something cooler looking. You'll need a freezer bag and ice pack to get the milk safely home.

Hand-Express in an Emergency

If you find yourself stranded without a pump, you can hand-express, which means using your hand to squeeze the milk out of your boob into a cup, bottle, or sink. It's not very effective or comfortable, but if you're desperate, it can relieve some of the pressure on your aching boobs.

Be Open to Formula

Daily pumping is a grind. Your supply might diminish when you're spending long stretches away from your baby. It's up to you how long you want to try to hold out, but if your supply can't keep up with what your growing baby is eating, introducing formula isn't the worst thing. In fact, it can be the best thing. It's an amazing load off your mind to not have to treasure every drop like a crazed breast milk hoarder. You may even decide to drop one of your daily pumping sessions or stop altogether. Whatever your interest level in the breast milk slog, it's okay. A happy mom makes for a happy baby.

Fun Places to Pump When There Is Nowhere to Pump

Another un-fun aspect of the on-the-go life of a pumping woman is trying to pump somewhere with no designated place to pump. If you want to make a statement about it, pump in full view of everyone. You can also ask that someone vacate their office or closet to make room for you. But sometimes you'll find yourself pumping in annoying places like these:

- A hot car
- A cold car
- A stinky bathroom while people outside wonder aloud, "What's taking so long and *what* is that sound?"
- Under your shirt on an airplane
- In the tiny airplane bathroom while people pound the door
- In a waiting room while a stranger locks eyes with you
- Random rooms that don't have a lock on the door that suddenly everyone will be very interested in exploring

No one has ever said, "I love pumping my breasts with a machine." If you can make pumping work—congrats, you're giving your kid a solid source of nutrition. If you feel like it's sucking you dry and want to stop, that's cool too.

FORMULA IS ALSO FOOD!

If breast milk is the nectar of the goddess, formula is the perfectly adequate nectar substitute that the goddess would nod at approvingly. If you're using formula or considering it, chances are that the mom-shaming environment we live in has you feeling some pangs of guilt. But rest assured, you're getting your baby fed, and that is perfect.

There are many reasons to use formula, but one perfectly good reason is because you fucking want to. It is not against the law to say, "Breastfeeding sounds fucking terrible and I'm not even gonna try." Let people tsk-tsk themselves into an early grave while you enjoy your boob freedom.

POWDER VERSUS MIXED

Some formula comes as powder that you mix with water, and some comes already mixed in bottles. For the first two months, you should only use premixed—it's safer due to sterility. After that, either is fine. Premixed requires less mixing but it is also more expensive and harder to transport in large quantities.

ORGANIC VERSUS CHEAP

You probably already know whether you're an organic girl. Some babies have allergies or digestive issues, which make certain kinds of formula preferable. As with many of these baby choices, we agree there are probably some qualitative differences between generic formula and the fancier organic kind. But if you're on a budget, the advantage is probably not worth breaking the bank. Like your annoying mom says, "You turned out *fine.*"

BABY WATER / INFANT WATER / NURSERY WATER

Some recommend mixing powdered formula with jugs of "baby water" from the drugstore, which contains less fluoride than tap water. As far as we can tell, most American tap water is fine for babies. Unless the water in your area is deemed particularly unsafe or high in lead, you can mix it with formula if you want to. This is yet another decision that depends mostly on your situation and anxiety level.

BABY BOTTLES

Some babies are picky AF about bottle nipples. Others DGAF. There's lots of conflicting advice about which bottles are best. We're sure you'll figure it out and your baby will eventually give in to not starving. Purchase as many spare bottles as you can afford. There's nothing like sorting through a pile of rancid bottles at 3:00 a.m. with a screaming baby in your arms because your partner forgot to start the dishwasher.

BOTTLE TEMPERATURE

Again, some babies are pickier than others, and over time your baby will care less and less about whether their food is body temp. To warm bottles, heat up a pot or bowl of water and then dip your bottle in and swish it around. You're not supposed to heat bottles in the microwave because the heat could scald your baby, but if you do it for a short amount of time, shake it up real good, and test the temp on your wrist, *whispers* *we won't tell on you.*

· · · · · · · ·

Like breastfeeding, bottle-feeding feels like a chore that will never end. But at least it's one you can share with your partner.

SLEEP: THE ELUSIVE WHITE WHALE

> Sleep deprivation is a literal torture technique, and as a new parent, nothing will make you feel so completely insane. If you have a baby who loves to sleep and self-soothes like a champ, this chapter is not for you. Seriously, GTFO.

their kid to sleep through the night the second they're born. Do *not* feel guilty that your baby is a rude, sleepless asshole. Babies are tiny and fragile and need a lot of attention. You're not weak or naive for giving it to them. Try not to strangle those making awkward chitchat about the bane of your existence. Many of them never had babies or already forgot how babies work. Sometimes new parents do this to make themselves feel better and to act like they have all the answers. They're likely exaggerating their successes and their baby is not *your* baby, so take any advice with a grain of salt.

"SLEEP WHEN THE BABY SLEEPS."

People always offer up the helpful but somewhat infuriating suggestion to "sleep when the baby sleeps." But this is easier said than done in the first few weeks when your baby is still nocturnal, bright-eyed, and hungry at night, sleepy during the day.

"HOW'S SHE SLEEPING?"

One of the most annoying questions you'll be asked as a new parent is how the baby is sleeping. The baby is probably sleeping terribly because they're a baby. While people are just making conversation, they unwittingly shame new parents for not getting

THE *ULTIMATE SLEEP-TRAINING GUIDE*

There are so many sleep-training methods claiming to be the best, prescribing what age to train and whether to do check-ins and what time you can put them down. If one of those works for you, great! But maybe you can't stand listening to your most beloved person scream their head off, or have a work schedule that means keeping your baby up a little later if you ever want to see them, or it's easier to cosleep, or your baby just doesn't respond to those methods yet. Here are our sleep-training methods:

The Simple Version

At whatever point you feel ready (most experts don't recommend sleep training until your baby is at least four months old), stick baby in another room at bedtime and let 'em cry for as long as you can manage; listen to your intuition. Rinse, repeat. Someday, they will learn to self-soothe on their own. It doesn't feel like it now, but you will get this. At first they will still wake up for feedings (most babies drop night feedings somewhere between five and twelve months), but eventually you will have a little human who sleeps all night.

An Alternate Version for the Rule Lovers

Wait two minutes. Stare at door for one minute. Open door. Whisper: "You're okay, this definitely won't scar you later. I'm a good mom." Shut door. Return and jiggle baby for exactly three minutes without pacifier. Return pacifier to mouth. Time how long between each crying fit. If time is lengthening, you are not a bad person. Send spouse out for lithium.

Feel free to read other sleep books and preach the gospel of whatever your baby responded to. But all parents and babies are not created equal. Some of us birthed beady-eyed, stubborn tyrants. We're not saying you shouldn't try to sleep train right now, because YOU + SLEEP = VERY GOOD.

Sleep Regression

This is when a baby who has been sleeping through the night suddenly starts waking frequently again. Sleep regressions often happen around the ages of four months, eight months, eleven months, and eighteen months and are often triggered by your baby's rapid brain development, teething, nap schedule changes, and any other big life changes. No two babies are the same, so if your kid's sleep turns to shit on a different time frame, just know that it is okay and normal and you may have your patience tested for a miserable week or two.

COSLEEPING

Cosleeping or bed-sharing is the practice of letting your baby sleep in your bed with you instead of in a crib or bassinet. This is a contentious subject because there is a lot of scary news out there of people rolling onto their babies in the night. Cosleeping is not for everyone, but done carefully, it is not the death trap it's made out to be. Some moms sleep better this way, since they can simply roll over to breastfeed and the baby is calmer with Mom nearby. If you want to cosleep, here are some precautions:

- Do not drink or take medications that could inhibit your ability to wake up or realize when you're lying on your baby.

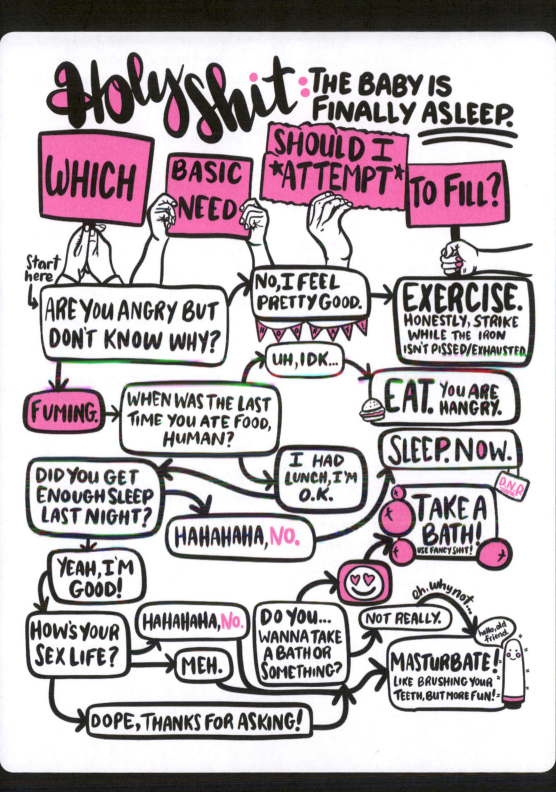

SELF-SOOTHING— WHAT IS IT?

Self-soothing is when your baby learns that you and they are not one person and they find ways to relax without being in your arms or on your tits. This is a tough pill to swallow, and babies find different ways of getting there with different coping mechanisms. Each has their own brand of mommy methadone, from pacifiers, to sucking on their hand, to cuddling stuffies, to rhythmically whining to themselves like something out of a horror movie.

Before your baby learns to self-soothe, they often need to be rocked completely to sleep, and if you put them down a second early, they will freak out like you dropped them in hot lava. As they get a bit older, you need to provide them with opportunities to learn to self-soothe, by putting them down to fall asleep alone, or not rushing in the second they wake up. They may not get it right away, but by not caving to their every whim, you are giving them a reason to grow and become more independent.

- Make sure your baby's head is not covered by any blankets or pillows and they could not easily pull objects like this onto their head in the night. Keep long hair or clothing with ties away from the baby.

- Make sure your mattress is firm and your bed is large enough (queen or king).

- Place your baby where they cannot fall off the bed or fall between the bed and the wall.

- You should be the one sleeping closest to your baby, since mothers (particularly breastfeeding mothers) have the most arousability and acute awareness of the baby. Over time, your partner will probably develop a better sense for this.

If cosleeping gives you anxiety, keep the baby close by in a bassinet until you feel comfortable putting them in a crib in their own room.

THE WITCHING HOUR

The witching hour is a time in the evening when your baby turns into a witch whose only magical power is being incredibly fussy. In the first few months this might involve screaming their head off for hours every night, requiring you to rock them in very uncomfortable and exhausting ways. Invite your partner to help ward off this black magic before it shrivels you into one of those small worms in Ursula's garden. You can also buy protective items, like a yoga ball or glider chair, to save your back from this evil and powerful magic.

SLEEP TOOLS

There are many ways to aid your baby's sleep, either by clothing them in swaddles or sleep sacks, soothing them with white noise machines, or placing them in swings, rockers, or other expensive products. What one baby loves, another hates. So try what you want and don't buy what you can't afford. See what you can borrow or buy used, especially if the raved-about item is expensive and seems like it might be snake oil. One benefit of not being able to afford fancy sleep gadgets is that you won't get your baby hooked on a drug you can't keep supplying. Because at some point, your baby needs to stop using the baby swing and learn to sleep on their own. Getting babies to sleep usually sucks. Luckily they can't be babies forever.

FINDING YOUR SLEEP GROOVE

Like so many aspects of parenting, you gotta do what works for you. If it's strict schedules and methods—go for it. Don't listen to the people who wanna come hang with your baby during nap time because "he can sleep later, right?" You're the one dealing with a tired, cranky, possessed baby, so *you* make the rules. And if some asshole wants to make lots of noise after you finally got the motherfucker to go down, because "you should teach your baby to sleep through this," that person can actually go to hell.

Conversely, if strict bedtime rules are more trouble than they're worth for you, you do you! Sometimes you can't match the will of a stubborn baby, and it's okay to let them sleep on top of you if it lets you finally catch some Z's for a couple of hours. You're only human. This phase will end. This is hard and takes time, so don't kill yourself with guilt over the imperfection of it all. You don't have as much control as some would have you think. In the meantime, we are sending you good sleep vibes.

SIGNS YOU MIGHT BE OVERTIRED

* You can't remember the names of actors, products, and everyday items in your own home, such as "soap" or "baby."

* You have vivid fantasies about murdering your partner as they slumber beside you.

* You find five breast pads in your bra and you only have two nipples.

* You go to grab your baby in the night but confuse their butt with their head.

* You're crying about something but you don't know what anymore.

* You incorrectly refer to your baby's name, gender, or the number of babies you have.

* You jump at every sound and hear phantom cries in your head constantly.

WEIRD POST-PREGNANCY BODY STUFF

Even after pregnancy, birth, and your semi-recovery, you may still be thinking, "This is my body now?" Here's some stuff you may be experiencing.

STINKY SWEAT

Your armpits smell like a stranger's now. As your hormones continue to fluctuate, you will find your sweat smells . . . weird. Actually, it's kind of the worst BO you've ever had. If you're breastfeeding, this may endure until you stop. Your hormones might be compounding this by amplifying your sense of smell. It's *strange*.

"BAD" HAIR

Many women find pregnancy changes the texture of their hair for better or worse. Leave it to the hormone fluctuations and that baby sucking all the nutrients from your body. While you're pregnant, your body maintains a constant growth cycle where your hair does not shed, giving you a pleasantly thick mane. But this catches up with you in a bad way a few months after giving birth, when you may experience constant shedding, covering your clothes and clogging your drain. This also results in some pretty weird baby hairs growing back in around your forehead a couple of months after that, as though you cut your own bangs very badly. We think it's cute on you though. Really.

SAGGY BOOBS

Breastfeeding might make your boobs look temporarily amazing, but at the end of the day, the swell of pregnancy and hormones might leave them a bit saggy. If you breastfed, your nipples probably look a little more chewed. All of this is okay! Remember, your body did amazing things and is amazing. Your breasts can be assisted with bras just like everyone else's. And if you never wanna wear a bra again because you've done enough in this life, we salute that decision too.

A STIFF NECK

The majority of your day is now split between two vertebrae-crushing activities: looking down at a baby and looking down at your phone. Curved posture and the weight of your increasingly heavy baby will leave your upper back and neck feeling angry. Fortunately as your baby gets bigger it gets a little easier to rest them on things. In the meantime, use pillows to keep yourself sitting a little more upright. Do some simple chin tucks through-

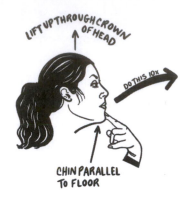

LIFT UP THROUGH CROWN OF HEAD

DO THIS 10×

CHIN PARALLEL TO FLOOR

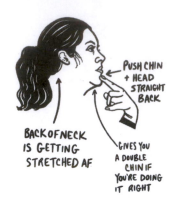

PUSH CHIN + HEAD STRAIGHT BACK

BACK OF NECK IS GETTING STRETCHED AF

GIVES YOU A DOUBLE CHIN IF YOU'RE DOING IT RIGHT

out the day, to help elongate your spine and stretch those tight neck muscles.

FAT FEET

As we mentioned earlier, feet can expand during pregnancy. Often they go back to their original size over time. But it may take a while, or not happen at all. At the end of the day, you may still be up a shoe size from pre-pregnancy.

DIASTASIS RECTI

Diastasis recti is a condition in which your abdominal muscles separate during pregnancy, leaving a gap. It looks like a ridge protruding down the center of your belly, sometimes only visibly popping out when you cough or sit up. This makes it hard to rebuild your core strength, and regular sit-ups or crunches can actually make it worse, so research exercises to gently strengthen these muscles, such as lying flat on your back and lifting one leg at a time. In severe cases, surgery is an option.

FOGGY MOM BRAIN

Turns out, there's a reason your mom could never remember the name of that actress. It was because she was remembering literally every fucking other thing to keep you clothed and fed and free of sharp objects. Add to that postpartum hormones and sleepless nights, and you've got yourself a mom brain, baby! This will wear off a little but probably never fully. So let go of the responsibility to remember the name of that person you met one time, or whether you met them, or even what day it is now. It's okay. You've got bigger fish to fry in keeping this kid alive. If anyone mocks you for not knowing meaningless trivia, laugh it off. They can be smug in their knowledge of nineties baseball stats or who Carrie Bradshaw dated in which season, but you've got a gorgeous little person. Your brain is still smart and good and all that other stuff is on Google.

HOW I LEARNED TO STOP WORRYING AND LOVE THIS BOMB BODY

Getting your body back feels nearly impossible with your hormones out of whack and a baby constantly attached to you. Go *easy* on yourself. You need to heal. You need to be realistic. And above all, you need to get some fucking sleep before you do anything else. Be patient. It should take at least as long for your body to go back to the way it was prepregnancy as it did to get you here (ten months), and it often takes longer because you're busy taking care of a baby, for fuck's sake.

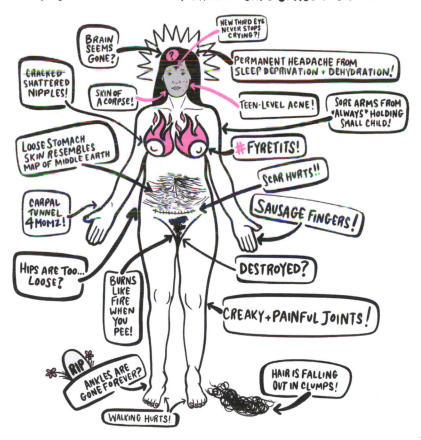

Gettin' It Tiiiight

If you delivered vaginally, things are stretched and will take a while to go back. It's okay, remember, this is what your vagina was designed to do. If anyone makes a comment about your cavernous hole, thank them for complimenting your adequate breadth. Don't let their inadequacy issues get projected onto your amazingly expansive vagina, and don't spend a second worrying about being small enough for their tiny dicks. Your vagina is good. It did a good thing.

Kegeling versus masturbating:

Wanna get your vag back—*for you?* You can restore the strength of pelvic-floor muscles with Kegels, which are incredibly tedious, or you can work those muscles the fun way—with masturbation. Sure, Kegels are a more sustained way of working the muscles, but you could also have *multiple* orgasms. Kegels *do* allow you to work your muscles while sitting in traffic, but they were definitely invented by a man,[*] who probably didn't think too hard about what those muscles are for, which is the female orgasm, dude! Either way, work those muscles and you'll be less likely to pee your pants when you sneeze, or pee your pants when you run. And best of all, you will have better, stronger orgasms.

Make Peace with the Extra Pounds

Some women lose the baby weight easier than others. Sometimes breastfeeding helps the pounds fall off. But some women actually gain weight while breastfeeding. Be kind to yourself while your hormones are still in flux. Ease into exercise. Make sure you're getting adequate nutrition for breastfeeding and baby jostling and healing your body. Try to find clothes that fit and help you feel good about where you are today.

HOW TO KEGEL

Clench like you're trying not to pee, then clench your butt like you're trying not to fart, then find the muscles that are actually *in between* those two muscles and clench *those* muscles. *That's* where the true Kegel lies. Get it, girl!

---

* Literally Dr. Kegel. Look it up.

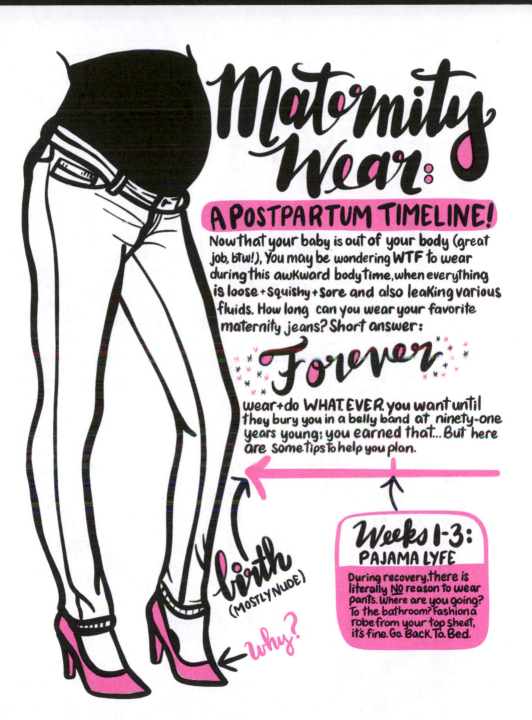

Maternity Wear:

A POSTPARTUM TIMELINE!

Now that your baby is out of your body (great job, btw!), you may be wondering WTF to wear during this awkward body time, when everything is loose + squishy + sore and also leaking various fluids. How long can you wear your favorite maternity jeans? Short answer:

Forever

wear + do WHAT. EVER. you want until they bury you in a belly band at ninety-one years young; you earned that... But here are some tips to help you plan.

birth
(MOSTLY NUDE)

why?

Weeks 1-3:
PAJAMA LYFE

During recovery, there is literally NO reason to wear pants. Where are you going? To the bathroom? Fashion a robe from your top sheet, it's fine. Go. Back. To. Bed.

Weeks 4-36:
NURSING CAMIS, YOGA PANTS, AND ALL THINGS STRETCHY!

Not nursing? Not doing any exercise, ever? No matter, Queen; Comfy clothes are your divine maternal right!

PRO TIP!
No time for showers or eyebrow maintenance? Kill two birds with one gross stone + comb that greasy mane over your face to camoflage even the Frida-est of unibrows! ♥

P.S.— YOU ARE PERFECT.

Week 36-death:
LIVE YOUR BEST LIFE!

Remember, boo: You made a person with that body, so love it, be kind to it, and wear WHAT. EVER. YOU. WANT.

There is nothing too short, too long, too young, too old... etc., etc., etc. Wear what feels good; anything else is oppression. Today can be the day you start living your truth + dressing like a middle school art teacher! And listen, if some dumbass calls you "matronly"? Look it up, that shit means Dignified.

6 Months:
PEAK BODY FRUSTRATION

Most women report that this is when they feel most upset with the state of their postpartum body. Be kind + patient with yourself; you are still healing. Resist the urge to try on your pre-pregnancy jeans; trust.

Week 4:
YOUR BELLY BAND HAS OFFICIALLY BECOME TOO LOOSE TO STAY PUT...

It's a strapless bra, now!

Week 36?
PANTS THAT HAVE A ZIPPER? MAYBE?

NO rush, though.

death
(MOSTLY NUDE, BUT FOR A BELLY BAND)

MORE CRYING!

> Your baby's not the only one crying. You may be unleashing lots of tears as well.

WHAT ARE THE "BABY BLUES"?

No, we're not talking about Chris Hemsworth's eyes, we're talking about those early postpartum crying spells that 70 to 80 percent of women experience and no one really talks about. Baby blues begin in the first days after birth, which feels pretty confusing, since everyone is congratulating you and saying things like, "You must be over the moon!" It's okay that you're not over the moon; that's a stupid euphemism anyway.

Science isn't completely clear on what causes these mood issues, because science can't really be bothered, because the patriarchy. However, most researchers agree that they are caused by a combination of the powerful hormonal changes that occur in a woman's body during these times and the incredibly stressful life changes that occur when a woman becomes a mother. Think about it: just a few weeks ago you had your feet up watching Netflix, surrounded by presents while people brought you snacks, and now you are the primary caregiver of a very tiny and fragile human being who hates sleep and wants to suck the life from your bones. Yes, they are very cute and you love them more than you knew you could love anyone, but good stress is still stress, mama.

If you get the blues, you may experience things like unexplained crying spells and feelings of depression and regret, irritability, restlessness, insomnia, anxiety, poor concentration, and fatigue. You may also have the urge to buy a slide guitar and begin composing twelve-bar blues songs. Feel free to follow this impulse. And feel free to cry. Crying helps your body feel good by shedding stress hormones and releasing endorphins. Don't suppress your emotions. You're feeling a lot, and it's good to let it out. The baby blues may come and go, or hang out for a while. If they last more than two weeks, it's likely that you're experiencing some degree of postpartum depression (PPD).

THE (INCREDIBLY FLAWED) STATISTICS OF POSTPARTUM DEPRESSION

According to the Centers for Disease Control, 11 to 20 percent of new mothers experience symptoms of postpartum depression. The problem with those statistics is they include only self-reported data from women who were brave enough and had the resources available to admit what they were experiencing. Studies have shown that women living in poverty and women of color are not only at a higher risk but also have more cultural stigma to break through, which is a very big barrier to care. From our anecdotal research (asking our mom friends), we believe that the true percentages are *much* higher. We tell you this to reassure you: if you are experiencing symptoms of PPD, you are *not alone* and there is help available.

When Does It Start?

PPD can begin at any time during the first postpartum year. Some women experience symptoms immediately after birth, and some are fine for several months and then start to feel like shit. Symptoms can by triggered by a variety of things, including beginning a hormonal birth control, experiencing increased stress, the return of your period, or beginning the process of weaning your baby.

"Do I have PPD, or am I just a bitch now?"

Part of the struggle to recognize PPD is how different it looks in different women. Common symptoms of postpartum depression look pretty similar to baby blues but are marked by their duration: more than two weeks of consistent symptoms of mood alteration, whatever that looks like for you. The words "blues" and "depression" are a misnomer; some women experience rage,

mania, and even psychosis. PPD (and all depression, really) can make you feel isolated and alone and unable to connect to other people, including your partner and your baby. This is a really scary feeling, and a very good indicator that it's time to reach out for help. If you're not sure if your symptoms match up, take the short quiz on the facing page.

Other Postpartum Mental Health Issues

While PPD is the most talked about, there are other postpartum mental health issues that necessitate treatment. You may have just one, or you may have hit the mental health jackpot and have them all! None of them are your fault, and all of them are treatable and temporary.

Postpartum anxiety (PPA) is characterized by excessive worry, insomnia, racing or intrusive thoughts (imagining that something bad is going to happen to your baby and not being able to shake the feeling or stop the images from playing in your head), and physical symptoms like nausea, sweating, loss of appetitive, and increased heart rate.

Postpartum psychosis is pretty rare and considered a psychiatric emergency. If you experience the following symptoms within two weeks of delivering your baby, go directly to the emergency room: severe confusion, mania, loss of inhibition, paranoia, hallucinations, and delusions. Again, this is very rare.

How Do I Get Help?

If you think you may be experiencing PPD or another postpartum mental health issue, the first step is to let people who you trust know. Tell them that you think you need help and have them read this information so that you can be on the same page. Reaching out for help is hard, especially when you are feeling so overwhelmed by life, and particularly because societal expectations make us wary of admitting that we are not naturally and effortlessly thriving as new mothers. *This is toxic bullshit.* You are a strong warrior who made a life, and your body is telling you that it needs help right now. Remember: your brain is just a part of your body, so let's treat this like we would any other illness. If you had the flu, you would go to the doctor. You have the flu in your brain, boo. You will heal.

Once you have filled your trusted people in, the next step is to find professional care. If you love your doctor or midwife (particularly if they have already briefed you on PPD and asked you to check in with them if you feel like you may be at risk), make an appointment ASAP. If want to find a new ob-gyn, ask some of your dope female friends who they like. You deserve excellent care. Don't go back to shitty providers, it only makes them richer and shittier.

When you or your support person call to make an appointment, you may need to tell the receptionist that you are having a mental health emergency in order to get in there quickly, and it's okay to feel embarrassed while you do that, but do it. Just say the words, they've heard them many times before. Here's a sample script:

Receptionist: Thank you for calling Vagina Experts, how may I help you?

You: Hi, my name is _____, and I am a patient of Dr. _____. I need to make an emergency appointment, because I believe I may be suffering from postpartum depression, and I need help.

Receptionist: *completely unfazed and just doing their job* Sure, I can fit you in on Wednesday at three p.m.

You: Thank you.

Receptionist: Sure, see you then.

You: *hangs up, probably imagines that receptionist is judging you*

Us (in your head): She isn't.

If you're not able to get an appointment quickly, seek alternate care. If you already have a therapist, call them. If you don't, search the internet for PPD resources in your area. If this is all becoming an overwhelming task for your already addled brain, ask someone to research and make these calls for you.

If you are experiencing suicidal or homicidal feelings, go to the emergency room right now.

PPD Treatment

Treatment looks different for different people. Getting on an antidepressant or antianxiety medication is a great first step that lots of women feel hesitant to take. Remember that this is a temporary problem with a temporary solution. Your hormones are messing with your brain chemicals, so giving your brain some chemical help will really help to clear the fog and move toward long-term changes that will make you a happier, healthier mother. Six months of Zoloft is a small price to pay for a lifetime of good memories. There are many medications that are safe to use while breastfeeding, so don't worry about that.

Many therapists specialize in the postpartum period, and there are many different modalities that can help alleviate the painful symptoms of PPD. Talk therapy is great for emotional stress and processing, and somatic therapy can be incredibly useful if you have physical symptoms like painful muscle tension. If you truly feel like you don't have the time or money, look for therapists who charge on a sliding scale, group therapy, a therapist you can Skype with, or support groups online. Whatever you can manage is better than nothing at all.

Stress relief and help from your community will also be vital to your recovery. When someone offers to come over and hold your baby, say yes. Take a nap, go for a walk, go to the gym, take yourself to the movies. Ask your partner to help you with night wakings; you do not have to do this shit alone.

IT MAY TAKE TIME, BUT YOU'LL FEEL LIKE YOURSELF AGAIN

Unlike some physical illnesses, mental health remedies tend to be a bit more nuanced. It may take you a few tries to find the right medication, the right therapist, the right self-care plan that gets you back to feeling like you. This is one of the biggest barriers to getting the care that you need, because depression already makes you feel hopeless and overwhelmed and *also* you are taking care of a baby, so the idea of having to try new things and be brave and face possible failures is a lot to handle. You can handle it. You will survive it, and you will someday be sitting across the table from another new mom who needs to hear this story to get the help that *she* needs. Welcome to the club, mama. There are so many of us, and we make one another stronger.

In the past week...

Circle your answer:

I have been able to laugh and see the funny side of things. →
- As much as I always could (0)
- Not as much now (1)
- Much less often now (2)
- Not at all (3)

← # OF POINTS

I have looked forward with enjoyment to things. →
- As much as I ever did (0)
- Less than I used to (1)
- Much less than I used to (2)
- Hardly ever (3)

I have blamed myself unnecessarily when things go wrong. →
- Yes, most of the time (3)
- Yes, sometimes (2)
- Not very often (1)
- Never (0) ← TELL US YOUR SECRET, QUEEN!

I have been anxious or worried for no good reason. →
- No, not at all (0)
- Hardly ever (1)
- Yes, sometimes (2)
- Yes, often (3)

I have felt scared or panicky for no very good reason. →
- Yes, very often (3)
- Yes, sometimes (2)
- No, not very much (1)
- No, not at all (0)

Things have been getting overwhelming. →
- Yes, most times I can't cope well (3)
- Yes, sometimes I can't cope well (2)
- No, most times I am coping o.k. (1)
- No, I am coping as well as ever (0)

I have been so unhappy that I've had trouble sleeping. →
- Yes, most of the time (3)
- Yes, sometimes (2)
- Not very often (1)
- Never (0)

I have felt sad or miserable. →
- Yes, most of the time (3)
- Yes, pretty often (2)
- Not very often (1)
- Never (0)

I have been so unhappy that I have cried. →
- Yes, most of the time (3)
- Yes, pretty often (2)
- Only occasionally (1)
- No, never (0)

I have thought about hurting myself. →
- Yes, quite often (3)
- Sometimes (2)
- Hardly ever (1)
- Never (0)

Total Score: _

RESULTS:

1-8 POINTS!
You may be experiencing the normal + awful mood swings of the postpartum period. Self-care time! If you still feel this way in a week, check in with your provider.

9-10 POINTS!
Give your doc a call; something is def. up! If it passes, great! Let's make sure it doesn't get worse.

11+ POINTS!
Congrats! You may have PPD. This may not sound like good news, but it kinda is. PPD is common, temporary, and treatable, but being a bitch is 4ever! Please call your doctor today and you will start to feel better SO soon. ♥

IMPORTANT:
If you picked one of these, please call your provider today. You are not alone; we have been there too.

YOUR BABY-CARE CHEAT SHEET

Besides feeding, there are other aspects of newborn care that may be foreign to you.

UMBILICAL CORD CARE

Your baby comes with a little brown stump attached to their belly button. Keep it clean and dry and leave it alone. You can fold your baby's diaper down for the first week or so if it's rubbing the umbilical cord. Do not try to pull it off, even if it's hanging by a thread. After it falls off (usually a week or two after birth), there may be a bit of blood or yellow fluid, and that's okay. Talk to your pediatrician if you see signs of infection such as a foul smell, yellowish discharge, redness on the surrounding skin, or your baby crying when you touch the area.

FINGERNAIL TRIMMING

Fingernail cutting is a seemingly mundane task that will somehow transform your sweet sleepy baby into a tiny ninja. Babies do not want their fingernails cut; try doing it when they're asleep. In the first couple of weeks, do not cut your baby's nails. Sure, newborns do scratch up their faces, but you could end up drawing blood, as the ends of their nails are still somewhat fused to their skin. Instead, file their nails or even chew them like a mama rabbit (neither of which will be very effective because their nails are tiny and flimsy). They sell little mittens to cover your baby's hands, but they fall right off. Baby socks stay on well but will require near-constant explanation of why your kid is wearing socks on their hands.

BABIES BARF!

Little babies barf everywhere all the time—on your couch, in your mouth, on your grandma at a funeral. Baby barf is actually not *that* gross in the grand scheme of barf. It's nowhere near as gross as adult barf. And you get used to it, sometimes anticipating and pointing the barf away from your shirt with the reflexes of a pro athlete. Other times, you just have to change your shirt for the fourth time that day. There is a lot of laundry. Have we mentioned people should be helping you?

DEALING WITH GASSINESS

When their little digestive tracts are learning to do their thing, babies can be sooo gassy. In the meantime you'll have limited success burping them, keeping them upright during and after feeding, and jiggling them gently for hours, perhaps while bouncing on a yoga ball.

CONTAINING THE POOP

You'll buy so many diapers. Get them shipped to your door so you're not lugging ten trillion diapers home while carrying a baby. Diapers are not foolproof. There will be blowouts. Especially early on, when their poop is basically a big bottle of mustard that they empty into an all-white outfit. If the pee cannot be contained, it's time to go up a size. You'll read the weight guidelines on the package and realize you should've sized up months ago. It's okay; you're tired.

You'll want to contain dirty diapers somewhere where they're not wafting in your face. Find an airtight diaper bin or put the diaper in an outdoor trash. As your baby's poops become more man-size, you may want to dump the poop out of the diaper into the toilet so you don't have grown-guy-size dumps hanging around in your kid's bedroom. But honestly that would require you walking over to the toilet, leaving your squirming child perilously high up on a changing table, so maybe just toss it into the bin next to you and call it a stinky day.

BATH TIME

Babies are *very* slippery when wet. They have no neck strength, so you'll struggle to keep their little heads above water while you try to wash them with your other hand. A good bathtub makes this easier, as does baby's increasing core strength over time. Babies don't always like baths. Try to keep the water warm and close to air temperature so that they don't realize what's happening. You don't have to bathe babies as often as you'd think. In fact, bathing too often can dry out their skin, so don't stress about daily baths. Be gross with us.

RIDING IN CARS WITH BABES

Putting your baby in a car seat for longer rides can be stressful. Once you're moving, they'll often go right to sleep, but stop/start traffic is a potential nightmare. Many babies have a hair-trigger response to alert them that the car has stopped and they will want *out*. Make sure they're fed before they go in, because there's nothing like listening to them scream on the highway when it's not safe to unbuckle.

HOW TO CHANGE A DIAPER

Put the new diaper under the old diaper before you open the floodgates. If things get ugly, it's more likely to spill onto the new diaper instead of whatever surface you're changing on, and both diapers can be disposed of with the destroyed diaper contained inside the other. If it looks bad, pull wipes out of the package *before* you unleash. You don't wanna mess with that tricky wipe dispenser once your hands are covered in poo.

The Tyranny of the Unplanned Car Nap

Once your baby's nap schedule has some sort of predictable rhythm, you get pretty attached to it. Baby nap time is literally the only time you have to yourself nowadays, and that time is *valuable.* Here comes the car nap to ruin your life.

WHAT THEY ARE

A car nap is an unexpected snooze in the car that disrupts your entire day. Sometimes they happen because you try to run an errand, pushing nap time a little bit too far back for your drowsy AF baby. Sometimes they happen for no reason at all, because babies don't actually understand what a schedule is or give a fuck what you'd like to do with your free time.

WHY THEY SUCK

Unless you've got one of those rare babies who will sleep through anything because you're #BLESSED, even the gentlest of transfers from car to house is gonna wake that baby up. And since babies don't wear watches or really understand the concept of time at *all,* they're gonna think nap time is over, even if it's been ten minutes. In a few hours, they'll be furious with exhaustion and scream at you, as if you purposefully engineered things to play out this way. They may even become overtired and refuse to sleep, which makes zero sense but is a thing that babies love to do.

So now, you're trapped in the car. It might be a short little catnap, or it could be a three-hour snoozefest where you have to straddle-pee into a Styrofoam coffee cup in your front seat; there's really no telling! Hopefully you have some purse snacks.

HOW TO AVOID THEM

Make sure you're home about thirty minutes before you know a nap is about to start. If you're headed home and you see your baby starting to get drowsy, it might be a good idea to start loudly singing, but nothing too soothing or pretty-sounding. Your goal here is to annoy your baby so that she is unable to succumb to the soothing lull of the car. "Are we there yet, baby?" you could ask her. She won't get it, but you'll laugh. Inevitably, as soon as you turn your attention to driving like a responsible adult, your baby will be completely asleep.

HOW TO SURVIVE THEM

If you're gonna be stuck in the car, you'll want to be prepared. Always have a car charger for your phone so you can endlessly scroll the internet. Keep a plentiful stash of adult snacks and drinks in your car, so you don't end up panic-eating teething wafers during a marathon nap that leaves you ravenous. What other things do you like to do? Knitting? Sure, keep some knitting shit in the car. Also, this book!

BABY FOMO*

Sometimes when a baby wakes up from an unexpected nap, they're super pissed.

* Fear of Missing Out

"Wahhhhhhh!!!" they scream, which we are pretty sure means "What did I miss?? Did anything fun happen?? This is why I *hate* sleep!" The best antidote to baby FOMO is fun, so if you had something cool planned for after their nap, like going to the park, drive there while they're still asleep. That way when they wake up, you can instantly distract them. Distraction is basically how parenting works forever.

WHEN CAR NAPS ARE ACTUALLY AWESOME

There are times when a car nap is exactly what you need:

* When you're pressed for time and far away from home, and you actually want your baby to take a little snooze so you can get on with your day.

* When you're taking a long road trip, and you plan your departure time perfectly and your child sleeps for the first three hours of the trip.

* When you have two kids, and they usually don't ever nap at the same time, but they somehow both magically pass out in the car and the silence is Pure. Bliss.

Don't let a car nap get you down, remember: someday soon your kid won't nap at *all*. Like, ever. Doesn't that idea make you feel exhausted? Maybe you should lean that seat back, lock the doors, and get a little nap in too.

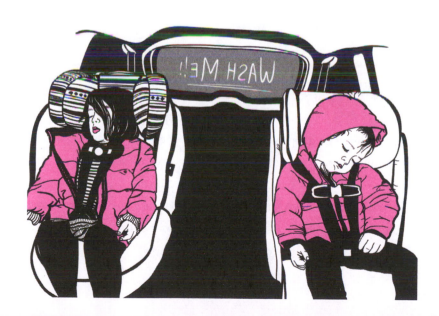

YOUR GROWING BABY

Your baby changes very quickly within the first year. Your tireless care gets more rewarding as your whimpering flesh ball turns into a chunkier, gigglier, alert human being. Here is a ballpark timeline of the baby milestones you have to look forward to.

TWO MONTHS:
SMILES THAT AREN'T FARTS

Somewhere around the two-month mark your baby will start to smile intentionally and not because gas is moving through her. The first real smile will make you feel amazing, even if those gas smiles were also pretty funny.

THREE TO TWELVE MONTHS / ALWAYS: TEETH PAIN

Teething seems to always be happening even though you can almost never prove that it's really happening. Your baby will just have a lot of vague complaints, fussiness, drooling, and chewing on things, which are all things babies do regardless. It might be teething.

Our world is strange and full of secrets. Whisper curses and buy some baby Motrin.

FOUR MONTHS:
GRABBING YOUR HAIR AND NEVER LETTING GO

Great news, your baby can finally hurt parts of you that aren't your insides, vag, or nipples. The aggressive hair and face grabs you'll experience while trying to feed your baby will make you feel especially "WTF, dude?!"

FOUR TO SIX MONTHS:
MESSY EATER

Finally, your baby can eat solids. On the one hand, you have to clean mushy peas out of someone's ears and their poo smells worse now. On the other hand, a baby in a high chair is a vacation for your arms and your mustard poo days are over.

FIVE MONTHS:
STRANGER DANGER

Just as your baby was starting to shows signs of independence, they've decided that everyone who isn't you is terrifying. It's cool; it's cool. You didn't actually want your arms back. No one will notice your slumped posture because they're too busy backing away from your shrieking child.

A Scrapbook That Won't Let You Forget

The cruelest joke of motherhood is how easily we forget the bad parts. This is ultimately our brains trying to protect us, but it also stops us from being as able to empathize with other women, and specifically with new moms. However, we aspire to a greater future, where no mom ever utters the words "I miss those days," at a new mother carrying a newborn and dragging a toddler down the street by her melting ice-cream cone. We can be the generation who remembers and tells the truth so that no mom feels alone when she's not queen of Pinterest. To combat your evaporating lizard brain, fill these out, quick! You're already forgetting more shitty stuff!

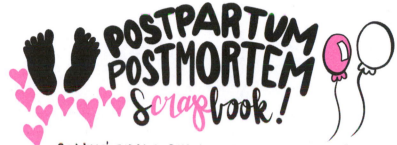

POSTPARTUM POSTMORTEM Scrapbook!

SO, WHAT'S THE MOST DISGUSTING THING THAT HAPPENED?

WHAT'S SOME STUPID SHIT THAT SOMEONE HAS RECENTLY SAID TO YOU THAT MADE YOU WANNA MURDER THEIR FACE?

YOUR BABY IS HERE! PLEASE DESCRIBE LABOR ASAP AFTERWARD, OR IDEALLY DURING:

DO YOU EVER WANT TO HAVE SEX AGAIN?

WHAT WAS THE HARDEST PART OF PREGNANCY?

DRAW A PICTURE OF WHAT'S GOING ON IN YOUR TIRED BRAIN:

HOW AMAZING IS YOUR BABY, THOUGH?

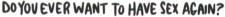

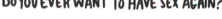

DATE COMPLETED: _____

SIX MONTHS: MAKING DEMANDS

As early as six months, your baby might say something that almost sounds intelligible, like "mama" or "dada." But we're pretty sure the sounds of "mama" and "dada" happen to be some of the easiest things for babies to say, and someone just assigned those sounds the meaning of "he wants you" when they were trying to hand a cranky baby back to a tired parent one time. Linguistics!

FOUR TO NINE MONTHS: CRYING WHILE SITTING UP

Finally your baby can sit up and, more important, cry from an upright position where they have a better view of all the things you're not giving them to put in their mouths.

EIGHT MONTHS: CRAWLING TOWARD THE OUTLETS

Now that your baby can crawl, they are finally free to pursue the most dangerous thing in any room. It's like a superpower.

EIGHT TO NINE MONTHS: CRUISING FOR A BRUISING

Before they walk, babies practice by "cruising" (using objects for balance as they walk). You'll watch with bated breath for their hand to slip and them to fall into things from a higher and more dangerous height than they've ever fallen before. These developmental leaps are so exciting!

COMPARING YOUR BABY TO OTHER BABIES

It's tempting to compare your baby to other babies to get a sense of what's normal and also whose baby is better. If you want to feel crazy, be sure to compare every metric, from head size to the amount of teeth. This way, you can feel terrible about your kid's slow growth. Remember, having kids is a competition.

How to Live a Tidy, Minimalist Life While Still Providing Constant Sensory-Development Activities for Your Child

* Only buy natural, wooden toys. Ignore their love of color, especially primary colors. They don't know what's best for them and their future aesthetic.

* Go "full Montessori" and provide your child with a monochromatic living space complete with floor bed, empty bookshelves (leave room for them to *imagine* the books), and only three ambiguous "toys": a spoon, a small wooden block, and . . . like literally just the next thing you see after reading this sentence is fine.

* Baby Kondo: throw out all stuffies that don't "bring your baby joy."

* Get a bunch of doorknobs and locks and wheels and other things you normally try to discourage your baby from fucking with, and screw them onto a big board. Now it's curated! Just explain to your baby that these ones are an interactive art piece, so it's okay to touch.

* Rather than cluttering the house with ephemera and photos, store *all* memories on the cloud. If necessary, take sleeping medication to combat nightmares about losing your data.

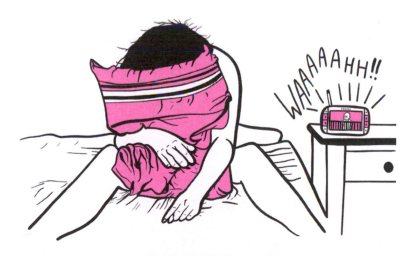

CUTTING THE BS OUT OF YOUR LIFE POST-BABY

A great thing about all the trials of parenting is that it truly does teach you how to stop giving a fuck. When your baby's health and happiness are on the line, everyone else's concerns are just noise. You no longer have time to obsess over your self-worth, some upcoming event, whether people like you, or your old perfectionist ways. So throw up your hands and rock shit like a mom. Here are some things you can stop caring about forever:

- Whether people like your kid's name/hair/face

- Whether your friend included you in her wedding

- Whether pulling over on this stretch of road to put the pacifier in your screaming child's mouth is "legal"

- Whether your friend's boyfriend is uncomfortable seeing your boobs while you nurse

- Whether you "seem scary"

While you'll care less about some things, other issues will turn you into an angry mama bear. Trying to protect the delicate balance of your existence is actually a great opportunity to develop the skill of setting boundaries. Sometimes stating your desires isn't enough and you have to resort to desperate measures. . . .

LEARNING TO MOM RAGE

You shot a human being out of your vagina and have gone weeks without a good night's sleep, so go ahead and yell at someone if you need to. This is your time to be a scary mom, so Live. It. Up. Moms each rage in their own ways and depending on the situation. Here are some options:

- **The glowering death stare.** Perfect for spouses when you need to make a point in a public place without causing too large a scene.

- **The throaty growl.** Perfect for the waiter who hasn't brought your drink for a half hour, even though you clearly need a drink more than anyone in the world.

- **The all-out scream.** When some idiot is trying to pull their car out toward your stroller, and you need to make your point quickly.

- **The pillow scream.** When you're home alone and the baby just woke up after napping for literally four minutes and you were just about to finally lie the fuck down for a second and a scream needs to come out ASAP. Let that shit out before you go in there all Zen mommy, by pressing your face deep into the pillow you never get to sleep on, and let 'er rip.

"AH, THE EASY DAYS!" AND OTHER THINGS YOU SHOULD BE ALLOWED TO CUT A BITCH FOR SAYING

Picture this: It's a hot midsummer day and you're pushing a stroller filled with a cranky infant, diaper bag, snacks, purse, toys, and water bottles. You've been walking for two hours trying to make a damn nap happen, and you're sweaty and thirsty and so hungry that you're snacking on Baby Mum-Mums. Your mantra: Must. Keep. Moving. If your baby doesn't nap, she won't sleep tonight, and if she doesn't sleep, you won't sleep . . . again.

As the sun burns your hunched shoulders, you see a family in the distance. Mom and Dad have large iced coffees, and Mom is holding a dog-eared summer trash novel. Both of her teenage children have working legs and do not need to be physically carried or pushed everywhere they go. They're talking and laughing and not screaming like they're being murdered by their stroller. You smile and think: "That's the payoff right there. The parents look so rested, and neither of them has vomit on their clothing! It's gonna get better."

As you pass each other, the mom breaks into a warm, dreamy smile at your screaming child and says, "Ah, the easy days! Savor it!" You look down as she passes, and notice her recent pedicure and then catch a glimpse of your filthy slip-ons, imagining the horror that lives inside of them. It's been a week since you showered.

Of course you will miss these days a little, but you also will not miss these days at all. Early motherhood is a marathon shit-show, and the cruelest part of the whole process is how quickly we can forget just how hard it is. Let us solemnly promise never to say any of these things to a new mom:

"Just you wait!"

Misery loves company, and miserable people love to tell you that things are going to get worse than they are now. This is usually not true.

"If you think you're tired now, wait until [insert looming milestone]."

Just when you thought you might actually get some rest tonight, another mom with older children appears to remind you that molar teething is coming. Or separation anxiety, or the dreaded 172-month sleep regression. Whatever they're referring to, it's usually *not* worse than having a newborn who still doesn't know day from night.

"You look tired."

"Thank you."

"Time for another baby, mama!"

Way before the last stitch has dissolved in your sweet, poor vagina, it begins. Once you have a baby, one baby is not enough. Perfect strangers will approach you to ask when you plan to complete your next miracle, because "he looks like he needs a friend!"

"Hello!"

Honestly people should just know not to step to you right now.

· · · · · · · ·

Remember: when people say stupid shit to you, they're either trying to connect with you and are not so good at that, or they're a jerk. Hormones can make it hard to tell the difference, and expressing yourself is the key to staying sane. Remember the advice of the Woman Queen of Planet Earth:* Speak. Your. Truth.

· · · · · · · ·
* Oprah. Duh.

DEALING WITH "THAT'S NOT HOW WE DID IT"

The cool thing about having a baby now is that medicine, technology, and various aspects of our culture are more advanced than ever. Like all generations before you, your child's life will be like nothing their older relatives have ever seen. They may be confused by it or bemoan change. Grandparents and other family can be very loving and helpful, but it's still okay to state your needs. This is an area where your partner should back you up, particularly when it comes to dealing with *their* parents. Here are some things you might hear them bitch about.

NAMES PEOPLE DON'T GET

Did you decide to name your baby something cool like "Satin" or "Chainsaw" or "Nosidam," which is Madison spelled backward? People will have opinions. Minimize their input by not announcing the baby's name until he or she has arrived. You don't need them trying to sway you while they think their opinion still matters. You get to decide your baby's name.

Your parents will quickly forget about it once they start spending time with baby Nosidam, whom they now can't imagine by any other name. If they're still making a big deal months later, we're sorry; they're terrible, but at least you've got some good stories?

DECISIONS THEY DON'T AGREE WITH

When you make a decision that's different from the one folks from older generations made, it tends to be triggering for them. It's as if you're holding up a mirror and forcing them to reconsider their earlier choices, and *no one* likes to do that very much. "You turned out just fine!" they will defensively yell, as you explain why car seats are important now, and it's not okay to hold a baby in your lap in a moving vehicle, "even for just a mile down the road." If you come from a tradition of circumcising or not circumcising, and then you do something different with your baby's penis, some people might be upset. Frankly it's a little creepy that they care so much, but it happens. Hopefully you can just tune out these opinions like the nonsense they are.

MAKING REASONABLE DEMANDS

One silver lining of the overexcitement of family is that you have a new power to wield over them. We're not saying your child is a pawn to be used in some petty mind game, but it is your right to command some basic decency from anyone spending time with you and your child. Reasonable demands include asking that your family refrain from substance abuse, verbal abuse, or any other behavior you deem harmful, such as the following requests:

- "We want him to grow up to be whatever he wants, so we don't shame him for playing with girl toys."

- "You can't smoke in here."

- "We want her to learn body autonomy, so if she doesn't want to hug you, she doesn't have to hug you."

- "We're raising our child to love all people, so we won't let you say racist things in his presence."

- "We're not commenting on her appearance like that."

- "He doesn't like when you do that. You're making him upset."

We know, it's hard. Trust us though; it feels *good* to set boundaries that keep your family happy and healthy and safe. If you have trouble saying no to your family, start with "Let me think about it," and work your way up to it. This gives you space to think and not be pressured. This is your family, and you get to decide how it works.

DON'T JADE

We all learned a valuable lesson from Gwyneth's GOOP scandal—jade eggs don't belong in your vagina, and JADE doesn't belong in your family either. When you make a decision for your family that other people don't agree with, it can be tempting to continue to argue your point. JADE is a useful anagram to remind you of what you don't have to do.

JUSTIFY—You have reasons, and you don't have to share them or why they are important to you.

ARGUE—If they feel differently from you, there's very little you can do to change their mind, and arguing will only send everyone into defensiveness. Do not engage with folks who want to argue with you about what's best for your family.

DEFEND—Speaking of defensiveness, it's easy for us feel defensive as mothers. The whole world has opinions about how we are fucking this all up, and that's their shit, not ours.

EXPLAIN—Say it with us: "We have decided this is the right choice for our family, thanks for understanding." The end. Mic drop. Tuck and roll and exit a moving vehicle, if necessary. You got this, boss.

BIRACIAL BABIES

If you procreated with a person or sperm donation of a different race, you'll probably end up with a baby who looks a little different from you and your family. Those close to you should approach your child with the wholehearted acceptance they deserve. If anyone is disrespectful to your child, either through sheer ignorance or willful hostility, go ahead and correct their words and behavior. And if necessary, cut them out of your life. You don't owe them anything. It is, however, your duty to show your child that they are loved and that no one should make them feel less than the perfect little person they are.

If your child is biracial, some DIPs* may assume you are not their mother. These are the kinds of people who also tend to be flabbergasted that your baby is a *girl*, since she is not wearing pink and does not have pierced ears or a bow in her hair. You can kindly set these people straight, and every time you do, you're making the world a better place for your kid and all their tiny baby peers.

If someone at the playground assumes you're the nanny, it's okay to laugh, because that's very ridiculous. Then say, "No, this is my baby, I made her. Isn't she just perfect?" If you're feeling bold/cranky, ask them why they assumed that and watch them awkwardly sputter and blush and eventually apologize while you sip your tea.

. . . .
* Dummies in Public

EMOTIONAL LABOR UNION WELCOME GUIDE

The Emotional Labor Union (Local 80085) is a group of mothers, doing the work of guiding other human beings through the world with the grace, wisdom, and comfort that (apparently!) only a woman can offer. This includes: telling your husband how to clean, telling your husband how to cook, and reminding your husband he is a father now. In return for your registration with us, we offer: camaraderie, reminders to outsource, and an unlimited text and data plan.

Your coverage and benefits will begin on the day of your child's birth, unless you have already been providing emotional labor to an eligible adult. Examples include: narcissistic parents, needy male friends, and codependent spouses. For a full list of exceptions, please visit www.emotionallaborersunion.com/whoiparent.

Depending on your coverage, you may be offered up to six weeks of assistance from a barely useful mother or mother-in-law. They are skilled at laundry folding but not soothing babies. Your coverage may not include emotional support from this caregiver, who may be triggered by this event in your life and need aggressive reassurance (grandparent jewelry) about your childhood. Please have your own trauma processed before this occurs.

As an emotional laborer, it may at times be expected that you parent your parents;

Emotional labor (n): the unseen and unpaid work of managing the daily lives and emotions of others, which is disproportionally assigned to women, regardless of their actual skill or willingness, as though it is an explicit function of their gender.

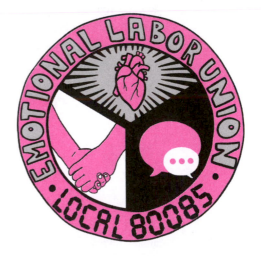

they need a lot of attention and thanks, and union members are expected to provide that service, in addition to parenting your kid(s) and also male partners.

If you are eligible for the family benefits, you will automatically be enrolled to receive harrowing insight into your own psychological issues and that of your partner. Please allow nine to twelve months for your relationship with your partner to become functional/pleasant again; the same timeline applies to your vagina. If you are not eligible for family assistance benefits, simply "sleep when the baby sleeps." Should be fine. You can also shower when the baby showers. Look, you were the one who wanted a family.

Please note: during the first several years of your new life, you will need to focus a large portion of emotional labor toward your partner. It will be your responsibility to burst his decades-thick bubble of privilege so that he helps you enough around the house.

Typically, our emotional laborers find that they are not interested in sex while tiny direct relatives are using their breasts as constant sources of nourishment and comfort; your situation may vary depending on how hot you think it is when your partner does the dishes once a week. We highly recommend masturbation during this time. Sex is a lot of work right now, and honestly where are you supposed to have sex when the baby's in your bed, the couch? You're a sweeter piece of ass than that.

Being a "bad mom" is grounds for expulsion from Local 80085. Bad-mom qualifiers are subject to change and additions at any time, but at the time of this printing were:

- Not reserving a #hashtag for your child before giving birth.

- Feeding your child sugar in any form other than seasonal fruits.

- Not practicing enough self-care.

- Too many plastic toys; so excessive and commercial.

- Too many wooden toys; who do you think you are?

- Posting too many photos of your children on the internet; you seem really lonely, are you okay?

- Not posting any photos of your child on the internet; your family needs you to provide them interaction with your baby so they don't have to ever put their phones down.

- Not exercising enough; don't you want to run around with your kids?

- Taking time for yourself to feed your mind, body, and spirit; don't you miss your kids?

- Cleaning too much, enjoy it while they're little!

- Cleaning too little; the children are watching you, and if you don't raise them in a clean space they will not love themselves enough to go after their dreams!

- Having a daughter who loves "princess culture"; what did you do to her to make her so basic?

- Not putting your infant son in a tutu ever; honestly how dare you assume he prefers masculine fashion?

Before your union membership becomes official, you must fill out the forms on our site at www.emotionallaborersunion.com/youredoingitallnow. There you will catalog the minute-to-minute emotional and physical needs of all persons with whom you interact on a weekly basis. Welcome and enjoy! Here's your membership pin! *Stabs you hard with pin.*

HOW TO NOT HATE YOUR PARTNER

Having a kid with your spouse or partner is pretty much the quickest way to fuck up everything good you had going. We're not saying you won't get through this, but you went from two people who maybe had to remind each other to clean up their shit and say where they liked to be scratched, to two people who now have a shared twenty-four-hours-a-day job that they are trying to manage with as little as possible impact on their former lives. Here are some relationship hacks for you and your tired partner.

Figure out how to communicate ASAP. There are times when one or both of you need to tap out. You both need to know how to clearly and thoughtfully express and receive news of each other's needs. Sometimes you need to tone it down in order to clear the air, and sometimes you need to scream at the top of your lungs so that your needs are met and you don't literally go mad.[*] Find a way to scream together effectively.

Find your systems. Maybe she does the wake-ups before 2:00 a.m. Maybe he empties the dishwasher first thing in the morning. Maybe you leave insane-looking Post-it notes around your home with memos like "REMEMBER TO ASK DAYCARE WHAT FOOD?!" Amid all the chaos, it's important to find some common threads to guide your efforts. Put it in writing or in a shared calendar. No one wants to find out at the last minute that their one chance at escaping for the week has been thwarted by "Dan's poker night" that he casually "told you about" over the shrieks of a child.

Get away from each other. You both need a break from your dark little stink den and each other's haggard faces. You need a quiet moment to check in with yourself with no one hanging on you or asking you about the person who hangs on you. So as soon as you're able, make sure you're getting some space, either alone or with friends.

Get away from your baby together. You need to see each other as peo-

---

[*] Remember: sleep deprivation is a factor in postpartum depression, so your partner should be helping you find time to rest.

ple again and not just the worker relieving you at the end of your late shift at the drool factory. Find time to do the thing where you touch each other and it feels good. Or if you're too tired to be touched, just eat a meal and talk to each other for once. You'll probably spend a lot of this time talking about the baby, and that's okay. Hopefully, this will help you remember why you two are a thing to begin with, outside of procreating.

Celebrate. Take time to congratulate yourselves for every little victory of your child's life. Whether they're getting out of the NICU or they learned how to imitate the sound of a burp. No one knows how hard-won these moments are like you two who are "in it," so turn to each other from time to time and acknowledge how friggin' incredible this little person is and how great you both are for making them.

JUSTIFIABLE REASONS TO RESENT YOUR PARTNER

Women are making a lot of progress, and hopefully your partner is stepping up to shoulder as much of the burden as possible. But being the keeper of the womb can stir up a lot of extra resentment, especially if your partner is male. The biological realities combined with centuries of sexist double standards naturally lead you to feeling a raw animal rage toward the man in your life, if not toward all men everywhere. Here are some totally normal reasons to hate him:

- He didn't have to grow or birth a baby.
- He didn't have his nipples chewed up.
- He is somehow able to sleep through that soul-piercing cry.
- He goes to the grocery store when you're stuck with a baby glued to you and somehow comes back without formula or the high-protein snacks your breastfeeding body is screaming for.
- He has the audacity to tell you he's tired after *you've* been in labor for eighteen hours.
- He gets to leave the house without worrying about where and when he's going to drain his breasts.
- He takes an afternoon nap like it's no big deal.
- He doesn't know where the diapers are even though you've had this baby for a month now.
- He tells you that you should "ask nicely" for his help with his own baby.
- He gets to go to work and have a life while you're still stuck with a baby.
- He makes himself food and/or drink when he gets home instead of immediately relieving you of the baby that's been on you ALL DAY LONG.

- He complains about literally anything in his seemingly magical life.

MENTUITION

[ment(y)oo'isH(e)n] (n)

A state of believing that you have intuition but making the wrong choice almost every time. The opposite of women's intuition. *See also: nontuition*

FIRST RULE OF FIGHT CLUB: HAVE A BABY WITH SOMEONE

Being a parent is stressful, whether you're struggling to make ends meet, carrying emotional baggage from your own childhood, or just trying to stay on top of the day to day. Managing it all with someone else is very, very hard. You're both tired. This is new to both of you. And no one remembered to order more wipes. Even the most balanced personalities will bicker while caring for a newborn, and most of us will at some point end up in a screaming match. That's fine. If it's getting to be too much, you may find the cost of couples therapy is very much worth it. You can get through this, if you're both willing to make the effort.

WILL I EVER WANT TO HAVE SEX AGAIN?

Do you want to have sex again? The answer is often a hazy "I don't know, *do* I?" Between your physical recovery and the terror of getting pregnant again, you may not feel very sexy. If you delivered vaginally, that whole situation is different now. And your baby is an ever-present third wheel. With the six-week waiting period bookended by late-pregnancy exhaustion and postpartum exhaustion, it's probably been *a while*. While you're the furthest thing from a virgin, you'll feel like one all over again as you try to remember the mechanics of it all. Here are some other reasons reinitiating sex might feel like a chore.

DRY VAGINA

Postpartum hormone fluctuations can make it hard for your vagina to lubricate. This issue can last longer if you're breastfeeding. This is your body's subtle way of saying, "Hey, maybe don't get knocked up because you're still feeding an infant from your body and life is exhausting enough right now!" Your body is so cute and innocent—it doesn't understand that birth control is a thing! Get your girl some lube.

VAGINAL INJURY

If you're still healing down there, you might not be ready for penetrative sex. Unfortunately you sometimes won't realize how uncomfortable sex is until you try. Establish a dialogue with your partner about proceeding carefully, and explain that you two are simply trying at this point and there is no guarantee you're going to want to see this to completion. In addition to physical limitations, a big factor in postpartum sex is your fear of discomfort. And fear is not going to help get you in the mood. So it's important that your partner is patient and gentle and understanding. You may want to do some solo play, or mutually masturbate, as you get reacquainted with your own sexual desire in a way that feels safe and low-pressure.

WEAKENED PELVIC FLOOR

The muscles down there might be weak right now, making it harder to experience pleasure or achieve orgasm. Do some Kegels or masturbate (see "Kegeling versus Masturbating," page 200) and you will slowly get your vag strength back. As a bonus, this helps prevent you from peeing your pants when you sneeze. But mostly, we do it for the 'gasm. Right, ladies?

EXHAUSTION

You're tired. So tired. That's okay. Sleep comes above sex on the hierarchy of human needs. Get some rest. Sex will be there for you when you're ready.

DON'T WANT TO BE TOUCHED

When a baby is on you all damn day, you sometimes don't have the resources to be touched by another person. The more your partner can take off your plate with household chores, baby jostling, and letting you get out and smell the fresh air, the more likely it is that you will be interested in having sex sometime in the next decade. The key to a new mom's libido is getting her a nice meal, a shower in a clean bathroom, and an hour or two a day where she is left the hell alone. Can you imagine?

· · · · · · · ·

Sex after baby is tricky. But you'll get back in the swing of it. After all, you and your partner aren't getting out of the house much anytime soon, so you may as well do *something* fun.

Birth Control: More Annoying than Ever!

If your partner is male, you're probably wondering, "How can I *not* get pregnant again anytime soon?" This might be tricky. Hormonal birth control has a risk of drying up breast milk supply, and tinkering with your already-sledgehammered hormones can lead to mood and body issues during the postpartum period (though some women have no issues at all). So you may want to hold off, use condoms, or get an IUD.

The risk of condom breakage might be too much for you with the threat of a baby so real in your mind. Luckily the discomfort of IUD insertion pales in comparison to contractions, and if your cervix has dilated from labor, it's easier to get it in there, so that's one option if you're looking for a long-term solution. Worried you might be allergic to the copper IUD? Wear copper jewelry or tape a penny to your skin like an insane person for a few days to see if you develop a reaction. Other IUDs do not contain copper but do contain hormones.

Talk to your provider about your options and your history of success with various birth control. There might be an unexpected solution like the birth control patch, which adheres to your skin for several days at a time and gives your tired brain a break from remembering daily pills.

If you're "one and done" (you don't want any more kids), a vasectomy is a great option that takes the onus of birth control off of you, which is awesome. It's literally the least your guy can do after all you've been through, and it will help to remind him how he witnessed your body be torn open to release his kin. Men tend to be pretty squeamish about the idea of a knife near their junk, but vasectomies are outpatient procedures done in a doctor's office and are seriously no big deal. Unlike babies, they are also usually reversible, if you ever change your mind about wanting another.

Reentering the world of the living after you've had a baby is tough. Whether you're squinting at the brightness of the world after you've been stuck inside for weeks or you're contemplating leaving your baby with someone else for the first time, it's often more emotional and overwhelming than expected.

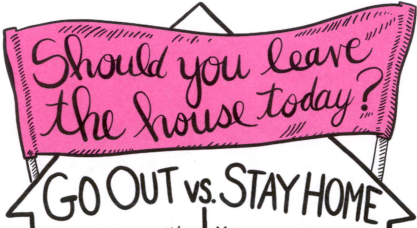

Should you leave the house today?

GO OUT vs. STAY HOME

MAJOR ANXIETY.	MAJOR DEPRESSION.
BREASTFEEDING IN PUBLIC.	BEING ALONE A GAIN WHILE BREASTFEEDING.
GETTING POOPED ON IN PUBLIC WITHOUT A CHANGE OF CLOTHES.	BEING ALONE AGAIN WHILE GETTING POOPED ON.
HAVING A PANIC ATTACK AT THE GROCERY STORE WHILE YOUR BABY SCREAMS INCESSANTLY IN FRONT OF STRANGERS.	HAVING A PANIC ATTACK AT HOME ALONE WHILE YOUR BABY SCREAMS INCESSANTLY AND ONLY YOU ARE THERE TO WITNESS THE HORROR THAT IS YOUR LIFE.
LACK OF SECURITY.	LACK OF SUNLIGHT, FRESH AIR, AND SANITY.
PEOPLE SEE WHAT A MESS YOU ARE.	NO ONE KNOWS YOU EXIST.

"WHY CAN'T I HAVE AN ADULT CONVERSATION?"

You know that feeling when you've spent the whole day working quietly, and when you try to speak your voice squeaks and crackles and fails and you're shocked at what a monster you've become? Well, after an extended period alone with a small child, something strange happens to new moms; talking . . . gets . . . weird? A little-discussed phenomenon, this side effect of early motherhood can really make you feel like you're losing your mind. Here's a good rule of thumb: after spending an entire day speaking slowly and lovingly to a very simple creature and no one else, the first adult conversation you have is a wash. Just let it be weird; it's always gonna be weird.

Sometimes it's a bank teller asking you if you're okay because you're stuttering and sweating from trying to remember what those "little paper things you put rolls of pennies in" are called; sometimes it's your spouse telling you about something that happened at his job and you just reply with "I don't know, what? I'm so hungry, I'm sorry? Do you have food?" Context switching between infant mother and adult woman is *hard work*. Go easy on yourself; you'll talk like you again someday. Your brain is not gone, it's just . . . napping. Maybe you should nap too.

BACK TO WORK?

If you're heading back to work, you'll soon learn exactly how much you love and/or hate your job. Nothing puts that into stark contrast like having a beautiful and demanding child at home. Leaving your baby can be scary, guilt-inducing, and sad. You'll wonder what they're up to, whether they're happy, and if their caregiver ever found that missing wubby. Back at work, things will be different and weird:

- You might be too tired to take on your usual workload and have to leave on time now to relieve whoever's watching your kid.

- You might feel pressure to act like you don't have a baby, even though it's *all* you think about, lest people start treating you like being a mom is all you have to offer.

- Coworkers might be constantly asking you about your baby or leave you out of non-mom discussions.

- You might be pumping milk during conference calls, or in weird sterile "pump rooms," should you be lucky enough to have a place to pump.

On the plus side, work has never felt like such a vacation. It's amazing how easy it will feel compared to dealing with a newborn. What a thrill to have a real conversation instead of staring into the void of feedings and back-to-back TV show binges. You'll be so relieved to be hands-free instead of being held hostage by a feeding baby while your glass of water taunts you from across the room. And while your brain might still be foggy from sleeplessness, you'll also find yourself more focused, more appreciative of your time, and able to get shit done like never before. That old saying "If you want something done, ask a busy mom"? That's you now. You're a pro.

NOT BACK TO WORK?

If you're not going back to work because you want to be home or because it's not financially viable, that has its own layers of joy, guilt, and shame. The cool thing is you get to see your baby change and grow. You get to be there for almost every precious tummy time, head lift, and sniffle. On the other hand, you have to be there for almost every tummy time, head lift, and sniffle, and that shit can get old.

Maybe this is exactly where you want to be in your life in this moment . . . and maybe you'd rather be anywhere else. As a stay-at-home mom, it's important to get out of the house. Find some mom groups, playdates, library sing-a-longs—anything to remind yourself that there's something out there beyond your doorstep. There should be cheap or free options in your neighborhood if you look hard enough. Just go somewhere. It's

hard getting your baby dressed and out the door, but every time you do it, you'll come home a little more capable and with a little more glint of vitamin D in your eye. And in between all that, put on the TV and let yourself chill the fuck out. You have the hardest job in the goddamn world.

STAY-AT-HOME-MOMS: STILL PEOPLE

If you choose to stay at home with your baby, please note that this does not mean that you're never allowed to go out without your baby. Being a mom all day every day is enough to make anyone go nuts. It will take a while before you're ready to leave your baby with anyone, including your partner, and this is normal. When you're ready though, you do *need* to learn to leave your baby sometimes. Sure, your boobs may swell up and you may text whoever is watching them ten times to make sure everything is okay. And at first you'll feel so much anxiety that it doesn't even feel worth it; but *it is.* Doing your own thing is the only way to recharge your mom batteries, so that when you are with your kid, you're present and feel good. What did you like to do before you were a diaper-changing, milk-producing robo-queen? Yeah, go do that thing sometimes.

Nanny versus Daycare versus Family versus You Forever

Here are some pros and cons of the various childcare options.

	PROS	CONS
Nanny	• Comes to you, so you don't have to dress and drag your little one out every morning. • One person devoted just to your kid.	• Most expensive option. • If nanny is sick, you may have no other backup. • You have no idea what they're doing all day unless you trust this one person's account or set up cameras like a crazy person (we get it though).
Daycare	• Cheaper than nanny. • There are multiple adults in the room if the shit hits the fan. • Your child eventually learns to socialize with other kids.	• Your baby will probably get sick a lot at first, which means you have to take off work to be home with them. • Your child gets less devoted attention.
Your Family	• Might be cheaper/free. • They might be more understanding if you're stuck at work late.	• Your family (or partner's family) is all up in your biz all the time.
Just You Forever	• You circumvent all the headaches above by never handing your child off to anyone.	• You may go literally insane.

Since our country gives new mothers about as much support as that flimsy nursing bralette, many moms need to find childcare before they are emotionally ready, so they can go back to work and afford things like food and shelter and the occasional almond croissant. Other women would love to go back to work because it makes them feel good and sane and like a whole person but can't afford childcare and end up staying home for several years because it "makes the most sense." Some women are able to make the choice they want but are still exhausted anyway. What do all of these women have in common? They all feel guilty about their "choice." Have we mentioned the patriarchy enough in this book? Are you angry yet? Because the idea that there are so many hard-working and hard-loving mothers out there feeling like they are not enough makes us want to burn.it.all.down. Seethe with us for a hot minute, and then let's shake that shit off and move on. Dig up the deep roots on those shitty feelings and plant something new there: self-love. Motherhood is hard. You are doing great.

ENTRUSTING YOUR BABY TO THE WORLD

Trusting a babysitter is an important and exciting mom milestone, and you'll know when you're ready for it. The sooner you can find someone you trust to hold your sleeping baby while you shower, take a nap, masturbate, sit in your car and stare at your phone for two hours, or even *go on a date?!*, the better. Don't let anyone pressure you into doing it before you're ready, and don't let anyone guilt you about doing it when you are ready.

It can take a tremendous leap of faith to leave your baby with someone who is not you. You'll want to provide a hundred-page thesis on how to soothe and nurture your demanding little one. Once you've laid out the basics—and this is very important—just leave. We know it's hard, but seriously, leave. ASAP. Get out of there. You'll want to call and text with "one more thing," but it's very important that at some point you try to enjoy your freedom. Sip the air. Run some errands. Get a pedicure.

If you're a chill lady who left your baby right away, cool! If it doesn't come easy, start small—take five minutes to walk around the block. Build up to a few hours. You can be you again. Not mommy you, but *you* you. A person with thoughts and interests beyond milk and cuddles. Don't get us wrong, cuddles are great, but the sooner you practice getting back to you, the easier it will be for those around you to support you, and for you to accept the support you'll need. You need it. This shit is hard.

MANAGING THE MENTAL LOAD

You shouldn't *have* to develop superhero powers in order to be a mom, but you probably will. Your new life requires a shift in gears. Some are temporary (e.g., diapers), but being responsible for another person isn't. For better or worse you're on call most of the time for another person's survival needs, and you have to adapt—fast. The name of the game is multitasking a.k.a. "the mental load." Some of your new mombilities will include:

- Pumping while breastfeeding while drinking water while checking your phone

- The psychic ability to sense when your partner is about to do something wrong

- Waking up and being instantly alert, multiple times a night

- MacGyvering a containment solution for a diaper blowout with one wipe, three diapers, a water bottle, and a T-shirt because that's all you have for some reason

- A constant awareness of exactly how much formula, pureed food, and/or Bamba is in your home

DEALING WITH MOM GUILT

Whether you're staying home or working, breastfeeding or formula-feeding, swaddling or freeballing, there's a way to feel guilty for every mom choice. The patriarchy pits women against one another so that we're constantly keeping score and measuring ourselves, and no one has energy left over at the end of the day to fight for mandatory maternity leave. Sigh. Women are coached into codependence from birth, so you've probably felt pressure to think only of your baby, even if it means turning into a hollow husk of your former self. Here are some things you're supposed to feel guilty about, but you *really don't have to*:

- Not thinking about your baby constantly while you're away

- Not being present enough when you *are* with your baby

- Having pleasures that don't involve your baby

- Letting your baby know what a television looks like

- Letting yourself get sick when you have a baby

- Looking at a cell phone when your baby is in the room
- Missing out on a potential educational moment for your baby, like pointing at a passing train and saying "train"
- Letting your baby eat a food that isn't nutritionally perfect
- Considering having a second kid who your baby would have to share you with
- Letting the sun get in your baby's eyes for a sec
- Thinking about yourself ever

Showering and Other Activities that Are Now Indulgences

Now that your life has been taken over, simple pleasures will be just out of reach. The silver lining is your newfound appreciation for these now rare and magical moments:

* Having time for basic hygiene routines

* Going to your job and getting to do work

* The miracle of modern appliances such as washing machines and Instant Pots

* Any moment when you're not holding someone

* The joy of sitting in traffic alone and listening to music without worrying if you're missing some urgent sound from the backseat

* The amount of food you're able to eat when a person isn't living inside your abdominal cavity

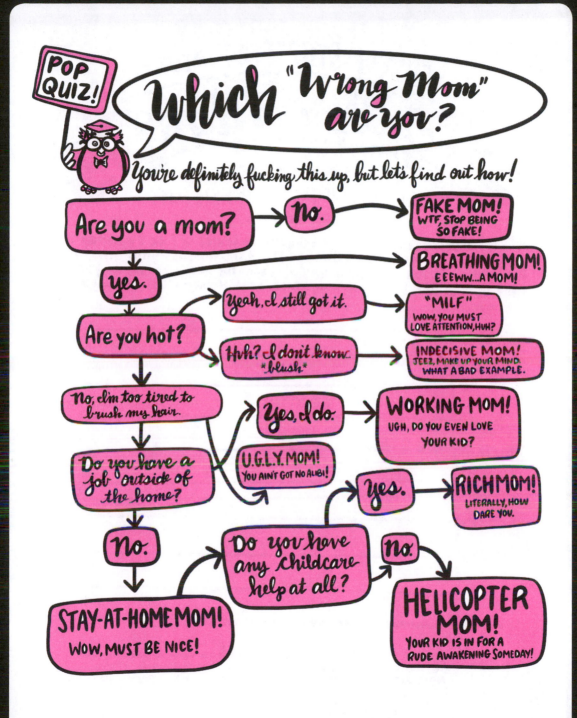

ALLEVIATE STRESS BY MOM-ING
Like a Man

WHY ARE MOMS SO STRESSED? BECAUSE WE TAKE RESPONSIBILITY FOR THINGS.

As you transition out of being your baby's main source of food, life, and overall comfort, you can de-stress by doing as the dads do—assuming that not everything is your responsibility! Stay sane by taking the easy way out from time to time and integrating more of these "dad choices" into your day.

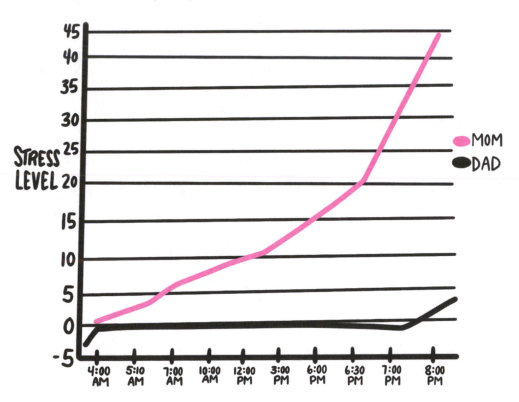

	Mom Choices	Dad Choices
4:00AM	Sleep fitfully, subconsciously aware of all that is to be done.	Sleep soundly.
5:10AM	Hear baby crying, rush to get up and comfort him.	"Didn't hear anything."
7:00AM	Realize you're out of baby food and have to rush to store before work instead of drying hair or looking in any way presentable.	Spend 20 minutes sitting on the toilet playing an iPhone game.
10:00AM	You barely got to work and it's already time to pump.	Read an article about the next Marvel movie.
12:00PM	Go to buy more pacifiers on your lunch break (where are they all going?!)	Go to Chipotle. Ignore the fact that you're sitting on a pacifier the entire drive there.
3:00PM	Pump again while working and also shoving food in your mouth so you can continue producing milk.	Text wife an annoying question you could've easily answered on your own.
6:00PM	Rush home to relieve babysitter while trying to respond to work emails at stoplights.	Go to the grocery store to buy beer without picking up any other food.
6:30PM	Try to figure out dinner while trying to calm a cranky baby.	Get home and turn on TV.
6:45PM	Give baby to spouse to change diaper so you can operate stove.	"Hey, did you forget to buy diapers?"
7:00PM	Shove food in mouth with untold rage.	Put baby next to spouse and walk away casually, wondering why she's in such a "mood."
8:00PM	Make spouse put baby to bed, and complain about his lack of effort.	Tell spouse she could "ask nicely."

Stop and Smell the Baby!

With everything on your plate, it's hard to slow down and appreciate the little things. We naturally want to get shit done and try to stay connected to the outside world via our phones, but looking back, you'll appreciate the small meaningful moments you had with your kid. Don't worry, you don't have to take them on a fancy vacay or teach them to read by age two. Just take a sec to connect here and there:

* Smell their head.
* Blow on their belly.
* Go under a blanket and laugh at the hilarious light coming through the holes.
* Go outside, or maybe just crack a window and tell them about trees.
* Sing "Row, Row, Row Your Boat" to them but change "boat" to "butt."
* Pretend their foot is a telephone and you have to take an important call. This works for *years.*
* Let them put their hand in your glass of water and watch their mind be *blown*.
* Show them your impression of a horse trying to hold in a sneeze.
* Press their face really close to your face and say, "I love you even though you're killing me."

F-You, Mom + Dad!!

SO EASY

An Easy Guide to Neutralizing Your Childhood Trauma, While Avoiding Damaging Your child in the Opposite Way!

YOUR DAMAGE	THE OPPOSITE	THE COMPROMISE
Your parents never bought you The art supplies/sports equipment/ taxidermic mice you begged for! As a result, you have not blossomed into who you might have been.	Buy your tiny, drooling infant any and all things they seem even remotely interested in at each bleary-eyed Target supply run. Never mind if it's age-appropriate (or even safe)! It's crucial (and suuuuper feminist) to encourage her early interest in power tools.	Buy her some toys, but not all of the toys.
You were essentially raised by "Sesame Street," and have no early memories that do not involve TV characters. You were recently devastated to learn that "Uncle Pee Wee" is not your actual uncle.	Zero screen time. Remove all "evil" screens from your house, and cleanse with sage to remove "negative ions." You may never get anything done again, but engaging with your child is much more important than a sink full of four-day-old dishes.	Talk to your Kid. Watch TV with them. Ask them questions about their favorite shows. Turn it off sometimes, and go outside.
Being an only child was very lonely.	Go FULL Duggar, stacking children on top of one another like precarious and expensive Jenga blocks, in every room of your house.	Have two kids. They'll be fast (forced) friends, and you probably won't need a Costco membership.
Your parents yelled at you a lot.	When addressing your child, NEVER speak above a whisper, and change your name to "Mother Whisper Wind." Scream into a pillow at night, for relaxation.	Wing it? Pillow-screaming is actually a pretty solid plan.
Your parents smothered you.	Leave your child to his own devices, even if that means flailing for hours in his crib. Did he ask for your help?!?! Jesus, Mom!	Ask your Kid if they are being hugged enough. Hug more or less, depending on their answer. If they can't talk yet, default to more hugs.

REMEMBER YOURSELF

You're still in there, you're just very tired. Find a way to feel like you, on days when you don't. The best way to do this is by doing something "selfish." Things that used to be mindless indulgences can seem selfish when you have someone else to take care of, but sometimes you gotta, even if you have a mounting to-do list and a mess of a life. So turn on that movie about dolphins you've seen ten million times, sit in a coffee shop and draw pictures of strangers, or go out with friends and eat a really melty cheese thing. All your bizarre little interests are what your kid will think of later as the things that make you, you. Model joy for your children so they know they deserve happiness. Seriously, they need this. So keep your baby alive and a roof over their head, but when you can, take some time to do your own shit, no matter how weird and unnecessary it might seem.

BUILDING YOUR CREW AND KEEPING YOUR SANITY

> It takes a fucking village, and you most likely don't live in one. Here's how to create your own sense of community in your new life.

KNOW YOUR PLACE

A well-positioned mother is at the center of the community that she makes, enabling her to be supported and to support others. Why is this important? Because when shit goes wrong you need people around you to help you deal with it, and when shit goes right you need people around you to celebrate with you, because you are still really fucking tired.

Archetypal Mom

This is the mother you aspire to be, an older woman who you look up to who shares your most important values. She might be your own mother or a woman who makes you think, "Damn, I wish *she* had been my mother." She is wiser and further down the road of motherhood than you. She doesn't need to be much further along the path, but ideally her kids are out of diapers, which means she's getting sleep and has time to think and return texts promptly.

This is the woman you call for advice when your child won't sleep, when you feel lost and like you're not a person anymore, when you need to find out how to get shit stains out of a wool rug. She has answers and the time to listen. She will remind you to breathe, that you're doing just fine and are amazing.

So how do you know who your archetypal mom is when you don't even really fully understand what kind of mom you want to be? Here's a good start: Your archetypal mom is happy. She loves and takes care of her kids, but she also loves and takes care of herself. She has boundaries, but she is kind. She raised (or is raising) children who are good people. She is thriving. The rest of it you can figure out as you go along.

Within the village of moms, you are also someone's archetypal mom. . . .

The Newer Mom

This woman is behind you on the path; she may be your pregnant friend who is due just a few months behind you, or your single friend who still isn't sure she even *wants* kids. To them, you are the wise woman. You have information that they don't have yet, and always will.

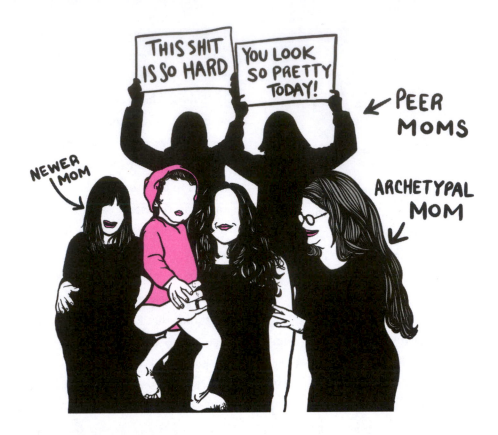

THIS SHIT IS SO HARD

YOU LOOK SO PRETTY TODAY!

PEER MOMS

NEWER MOM

ARCHETYPAL MOM

When a newer mom asks you for advice, take a minute to recall the stage she is currently in before responding. While pregnancy nausea may seem trivial now, as you battle sleep deprivation and weaning hormonal fluctuations, you've been there, and it was awful. Harness compassion—she has no idea what she's in for, and really, don't tell her. Remember how it felt when older ladies would say shit like, "Oh, just you wait!"? Let's let that gem die with the older ladies.

If you have a newer mom under your wing, make sure to tell her that she can always reach out if she's feeling depressed. Everyone deserves someone they know they can be honest with, and you can be that person, even if you've never been depressed yourself.

Peer Moms

There's one thing the archetypal mom can't do for you, and that's commiserate. With time comes wisdom and a broader perspective, but it also tends to scrub your memory a little too clean of the darkness and overwhelming feelings that are a very real part of early motherhood. So when your archetypal mom leaves you feeling a little less understood than you hoped, call on the peer moms.

Peer moms have kids in the same age group as your kids, give or take a few developmental stages, and they're about as sleepless and crazed as you are. They say things like, "No advice, but I'm sending you hugs," and "Ugh, girl, same." They can offer experimental fixes for teething and sleep regressions that they recently tried, and they probably won't work the same way for you but you'll be grateful anyway. They usually have a bunch of baby clothes they're giving away, and some different kinds of bottles for your baby to reject. When you text them at 1:00 a.m. and hope you're not waking them, you're not.

All of these women in your life serve a very important purpose. Your archetypal mom shows you that there is indeed life after baby, your peer moms are a daily reminder that life with a baby is good even when it feels like it will break you, and the newer moms remind you of just how far you've come. You may have one of each, or you may have a huge community of women around you, but remember: be choosy with who you add to your inner circle. Your time is valuable, and you are dope. Surround yourself with women who lift you up, because motherhood is hard,

and you don't need to make it any harder by having people around you who drain your energy or make you feel like shit.

WHERE TO FIND YOUR MOMS

Best-case scenario: You're all set. You and all of your friends have been carefully orchestrating this shit for years, and you have all purchased adorable and affordable tiny houses on the same street, overlooking both the ocean and also a bustling and diverse downtown. You're all pregnant together, and everyone's husbands get along. Good for you, go ahead and skip to the next section, you lucky . . . lady.

For most of us, community is a hard thing to cultivate as adults. When we pair off, life and jobs and family obligations take us very far from our friends, and then suddenly we have a baby to take care of and no one around who gets it. Hopefully you took our damn advice and took a prenatal yoga class while you were pregnant and met some mom friends there. If not, take a postnatal one, or really any sort of gathering for women who are new mothers: La Leche League meetings if you love talking about your boobs, mothering circles if you love patchouli-scented things, Mommy and Me at the local Romp-and-Roll if you love the smell of cleaning solution and the sound of shrieking; find some meetup for new moms and talk to all of them.

The new moms you meet will all be different from you, and this is good! Some of them will be annoying (avoid these), but others will be funny and honest and you'll get those weird butterflies like you have a crush, because new motherhood makes us all very awkward. The awkward first-date feeling is a pretty good sign that you have a new mom friend. Keep doing this until you've built a solid coven, and then start studying the dark arts together! Or, you know, have playdates. Up to you.

BUT, GUYS, I HATE PEOPLE

In-person hangs not really your jam, because you are super introverted right now and/or have a communicable disease? Start with online communities, and maybe work your way up. If there were ever a time to get over your shyness, it's now. You need all the support you can get from people who get it. And finding a community online is not that foreign a concept to modern moms. Need to find a sitter in the nabe you just moved to? Ask your local mom group! Up at 3:00 a.m. wondering if you should take your coughing baby to the ER? Somewhere some mom is online and ready to answer. But like the rest of the internet, online mom spaces are often filled with sad people with nothing better to do than try to cut other women down. So choose your groups carefully and try to remember you can easily walk away from a group or thread that's gone sour. If you're not finding what you're looking for, consider starting your own group and keeping it small and friendly. There are plenty of people out there dealing with the same struggles as you, if you're willing to find them.

Try to stay open to women who seem super different from you—if nothing else, they'll make you laugh when they sleepily text you a random GIF by accident. No woman is an island, but early motherhood can feel like being stranded on one, which is way more fun if you have a BFF there with you.

NON-MOM SUPPORT

There are also going to be people out there who are not moms but can still support you in everyday ways. It's important to lean on these people now. You need all the help you can get, and your mom friends are too busy to supply all of it.

Childless Friends

A lot of them might not appreciate your new hours, and some of them will turn out to be downright useless, but they can still be cool to have around, even if less frequently than before.

Mom Tinder—When to Swipe Left on a Mom Friend

While a good mom friend is an oasis in a desert of sleep deprivation and baby talk, a bad or toxic one is . . . what's a bad thing to have in a desert? Salty snacks? She's a salty-ass snack. Just as all salty snacks are delicious, all mothers are valid humans worthy of love and respect, but that doesn't mean you should be their BFF. Below are a couple types of moms you should probably avoid for your own sanity.

CLEARLY FRONTIN' MOM/ MULTILEVEL-MARKETING- SCHEME MOM

If she tells you she's not struggling while her left bloodshot eye twitches to the rhythm of her baby's cries, back away slowly. She's either lying to you or herself, and neither bodes well for friendship. Also, don't buy those pills/oils/leggings she's selling.

SPIRALING MOM

If this woman is already your friend, help her, but don't make a new friend who needs help/hates her life while you're a new mom. As women, it's easy for us to feel like it's our job to take care of everyone, but it isn't, and you need to protect yourself. New moms need support and healthy relationships. A spiraling mom needs them too, but say it with us: she is not your responsibility.

JUDGMENTAL MOM

As we all know from being horribly insecure teenagers, the lure of the mean girl is strong when you're the new kid in town, especially when she picks you to confide in. At first the judgmental mom may seem funny and honest, but pretty soon you'll realize she's not very honest about herself, and her "honesty" is really just an excuse to shit on other moms for their choices in order to feel validated about her own. You can tell she's gearing up to be judgy because she will start with a qualifier, such as "Honestly, I'm not trying to be mean, but . . ." This is when she's about to be mean. She'll follow with an opinion she has, stated as an obvious fact. Honestly, she's not trying to be mean, "but anyone who eats Paleo has an eating disorder." And "Let's be real, if you breastfeed your baby for more than a year, you're creepy." A judgmental mom is a straight-up bully.

There are judgmental people everywhere, so the judgment can take many different forms. She might put down moms for the way they dress, or their choice to sleep-train their baby, or their choice to not sleep-train their baby; the common denominator is that she's picking on people who are different from her, and that sucks. Motherhood is hard work, and we need to lift one another up, not pull one another down. Hard pass.

What They Won't Understand

- The meaning of "child-friendly" activities

- The preciousness of your time

- How very, very tired you are and why you can't meet up at 10:00 p.m.

What They Will Understand

- How to take you back to a time from before you were a mom, by doing non-mom stuff with you

- How to talk about culture and the world outside of motherhood

- Who you are outside of being a mom

Try to stay in touch with friends at least a little. Group text will save your life and make you feel like you're still a part of things when you're in the loneliest stages of your baby's infancy. Even if you throw out the occasionally passive-aggressive text about how "that party looks fun; I've just been marinating in baby barf over here," you'll be connected, and they'll have a better sense of where your head's at these days.

Your Family

If you have family living close by who you don't want to murder as soon as you set eyes on them, they can be very helpful. Find a thing they're good at or at least okay at and ask them to do it for you. This could be childcare or cooking or making your TV work. If it's a thing that could help you right now, you should ask for it, as long as you're being respectful and appreciative of their time and energy.

People You Pay to Do Stuff

We're not all Daddy Warbucks, but if you have a little cash on hand to throw at your problems, it's worth lightening the load, especially if your other support systems are lacking. If you can afford to, pay people who save you time and make you feel good. Every little bit helps make you a slightly more rested mama. Here are some examples of people you can gladly give your money to:

- Therapists

- Housekeepers

- Babysitters

- Food-delivery People

- Cabdrivers

- Spa and Beauty Professionals

Whether you have the money to pay people or not, a good skill to cultivate now that you're a mom is learning to be comfortable asking for help and accepting help that is offered. You need all the help you can get, and it is a unique burden in our society that so little of that help is built into our communities. It sucks that you have to reach out when you already have so much on your plate, but do yourself a favor and get what you can. You need a fucking break.

EPILOGUE: YOU'RE FUCKING INCREDIBLE

One last reminder before we close out this book. You and your body and your baby are fucking incredible. Really. Truly. You're doing an amazing thing. Sometimes it sucks, but one way or another, you are doing it. You got this!

We love babies, and we especially love our own babies. But keeping them healthy and happy is hard. Very hard. But it's worth it, despite the long bitch sesh that comprised this entire book.

You are *making a person,* from your own cells. That little person has light inside of them; they are pure good. You made that happen. You knit their fucking circulatory system with your mind, wizard. Those weird giggles are because you gave them a voice. The person you made is pure love, and you did that. Your bones moved to make room for them inside of you. Your blood rerouted, most of your internal organs stuffed themselves around your heart so that they could grow. Your body knew exactly what to do, and it still does. Your bigger belly, your wider hips, your stretch marks, your weird baby hairs regrowing out of the front of your hairline like an awkward fuzzy crown—these are all medals of honor. By the time you're through this shocking phase of early motherhood, you will have been to the edges of your being, and you will have brought someone new and perfect and beautiful back with you. You are a magical fucking creature.

WHY THE PATRIARCHY WANTS MOTHERHOOD TO STAY UNCOOL

You are literally creating life on this planet and that makes the male-dominated "powers that be" jealous and scared. The world would rather tear you down for not being a size zero and pureeing your own organic baby food than see how truly powerful you are. Since they don't want to give credit where credit is *overdue,* we'll say it again and again: You are incredible. Embrace it. Remind yourself. Especially when people around you aren't.

Few people work as hard as moms. So embrace the other moms out there. Nod to one another like veterans of a great and mysterious war. We're doing this. We can use all the help we can get, but at the end of the day, we got this.

You got this.

It's time to look forward because there is no looking back. You're a mom now. And that is something to be *proud* of. Congrats!

We're sending you all the love on
this magical journey,

Beth and Jackie

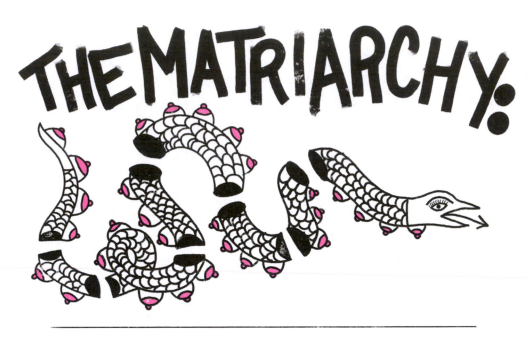

THE MATRIARCHY.

JOIN, or DIE.

ACKNOWLEDGMENTS

Thank you to:

Our moms Terry Newell and Ann-Marie Stone for birthing us, Peter McNerney, Alison Newell, Michelle Chiafulio, Kathleen Brimlow, Nancy Giglio, Alice McClain, Gina Mauro, Marie Funk, Silvie Falschlunger, Dee Yergo, Michelle McCoy, Hannah Adams Burke, Vanessa Kelly, Krishonda Washington, Amie Arbuckle, Josie Davis, Ashley Hawkins, Ashley Valo, Jarman Fargalde, Juliette Gomez, Jenny Caraher, Jennifer Jackson, Anais Murphy, Lauren Healy-Flora, Libby Sentz, Kathryn Merry, Maya Nardone, Mara Bernstein, Sarah Occident, Sara Pecora, Emma Assin, Melissa Otley, Stephanie Marte, Carolyn Noonchester, Miellyn Fitzwater Barrows, Kathleen Doyle, and the whole pile of moms who've helped and inspired us.

NOTES

1. J. M. Schlaeger, E. M. Gabzdyl, J. L. Bussell, N. Takakura, H. Yajima, M.Takayama, and D. J. Wilkie, "Acupuncture and Acupressure in Labor," *Journal of Midwifery & Women's Health* 62, no. 1 (January 2017): 12–28.

2. E. Burns, C. Blamey, S. J. Ersser, A. J. Lloyd, and L. Barnetson, "The Use of Aromatherapy in Intrapartum Midwifery Practice an Observational Study," *Complementary Therapies in Nursing & Midwifery* 6, no. 1 (February 2000): 33–4.

3. U. Bingel, V. Wanigasekera, K. Wiech, R. Ni Mhuircheartaigh, M. C. Lee, M. Ploner, and I. Tracey, "The Effect of Treatment Expectation on Drug Efficacy: Imaging the Analgesic Benefit of the Opioid Remifentanil," *Science Translational Medicine* 3, no. 70 (February 2011): 70ra14.

4. B. K. Alexander, R. B. Coambs, and P. F. Hadaway, "The Effect of Housing and Gender on Morphine Self-Administration in Rats," *Psychopharmacology* 58, no. 2 (July 1978): 175–9.

INDEX

condoms, 229

conjunctivitis, 140–41

constipation, 9, 20

contractions, 77, 124, 126–27

cosleeping, 192, 194

CPM. *See* certified professional midwife

cramping, 9, 123, 145–46

crib bumpers, 68

crowning, 129

crying

during pregnancy, 62, 74–75

postpartum, 203–7

baby's, 166–67

D

daycare, 233

deli meat, 21

dental care, 20

diapers, 67, 70, 209

diarrhea, 123

diastasis recti, 111, 198

dilation, 127–28

doctors, 26, 28–29, 114

documentation

of birth, 45, 94, 135

scrapbook as, 213

doula, 104, 114–15

dreams, 41

drugs

during pregnancy, 24

during delivery, 85–86, 95–100

recreational, 24

side effects of, 99

due date, 49, 80, 120

E

early labor, 127

eating

during pregnancy, 21, 40, 121

breastfeeding and, 183

emotions, 73–75, 166

Emotional Labor Union, 222–24

engorgement, 176, 178

epidural, 96–97

EPI-NO (device), 76

episiotomy, 29

essential oils, 108–9

exercise(s)

during pregnancy, 18–20

while preparing for birth, 78–79

after delivery, 157–58, 198

Kegel, 200

Expecting Better: Why the Conventional Pregnancy Wisdom Is Wrong—and What You Really Need to Know (Oster), 36

eye ointment, 140–41

F

family

asking for help from, 248

as members of birth team, 115–16

visiting after delivery, 161–62

fatigue, 24–25

"fed is best," 80

feeding, 169

feet, 60, 198

fingernail trimming, 208

first trimester, 9–14

floppy belly, 146

flushing, 123

foods, 21

formula feeding, 170, 189–90

frankincense, 108

friends
    as members of birth team,
      115–16
    visiting after delivery, 161–62

fundal height, 80

G

Gaskin, Ina May, 36, 107

gassiness, 208

gender reveals, 49

geriatric pregnancy, 81

guilt, 235–36

H

hair, 197

hand-expressing milk, 178

health care, 150–51

heartburn, 40

helicopter mom, 237

hemorrhage, 91

hemorrhoids, 145

high-risk pregnancy, 30–31

history of birth, 4–5

home birth
    benefits of, 88–90
    choosing, 88–89
    pain management during, 91
    preparation for, 91–93
    risks of, 90–91

hospital bag, 94, 117–19

hot flash, 62

I

ibuprofen, 147–48

ice, 93

immunization, 142

Ina May's Guide to Childbirth (Gaskin), 36

induction methods, 95, 100–4, 120–22

IUD (intrauterine device), 229

J

jaundice, 171

K

Kegel exercises, 200

L

labial tears, 144

labor
    back, 130
    best positions for, 134–37
    experiences during, 130–32
    signs of, 123–24
    stages of, 127–29

La Leche League, 174

latch, achieving a good, 177

lavender oil, 93, 108

letdown, 176, 178

linea nigra, 41

listeria, 21

T

TAP block, 110, 112

tearing, 144

teeth, 20

teething, 70

testing, 32–33

third trimester, 59–65

thirst, 9

toilet, sitting on to relieve discomfort, 131

transition, 127–28

U

umbilical cord, 38, 113, 140–41, 208

uterus, 38

V

vaccines, 142

vaginal birth, 144

vaginal discharge, 123–24

vaginal stretching, 76

vasectomy, 229

VBAC (vaginal delivery after cesarean), 95

vernix, 141

video, 135

visions, 132

visualization, 106

vitamin K, 142

vitamins, 22–23

vomiting

   during pregnancy, 8

   during labor, 123

   baby's, 208

W

walker, for baby, 68

walking, benefits of, 106, 121

water

   breaking, 124

   for hydration, 24, 131, 152, 174

   for pain relief, 53, 105, 121

weaning, 182, 184–85

weight, 47

witch hazel, 147

work, returning to, 231–32

Y

yoga, 19, 78–79

yoga ball, 94, 104

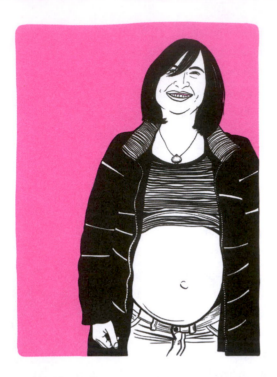

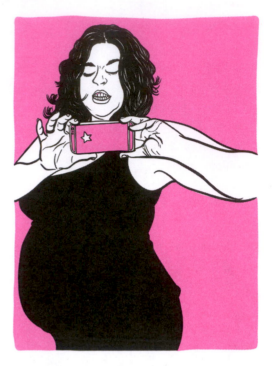

Beth Newell is the cofounder and editor of the satirical women's magazine *Reductress*. She coauthored the book *How to Win at Feminism*. Her work has been featured in *The Onion, McSweeney's,* and *The New Yorker*. She hosts the podcast *We Knows Parenting* along with her husband, Peter McNerney. Beth was named by *Rolling Stone* as one of the "50 Funniest People Right Now" and as one of *Time* magazine's "23 People Who Are Changing What's Funny Right Now." She gave birth to her daughter in the backseat of a Honda Fit.

Jackie Ann Ruiz is a writer, illustrator, mother, and performer. A native New Yorker, she cohosted the podcast *Best Friends, However* with Eliot Glazer and performed at BAM and UCB before relocating to Richmond, Virginia, with her family. Jackie is a resident artist at Studio Two Three in Richmond, where she works on commissioned illustration projects and is developing a coloring book for disgruntled women. Once an editor for a men's lifestyle website covering topics such as "Blue Balls Really Is a Thing," Jackie is now an out-of-the-closet feminist who is thrilled to be using her platform as a writer and illustrator to describe the harrowing and transcendent experience of pregnancy, labor, and motherhood, which changed her life in the best and worst of ways. Plus, she got to draw a lot of vaginas on her iPad. By the time you read this, she will be happily divorced.